The Elderly

Reflections from Family Practice and Ethics

Design & layout by Kite Group
www.kitegroup.com.mt
info@kitegroup.com.mt

First Published in 2025 by Kite Group, Malta.

The metal sculptures featured on the front and back covers were created by the author using scrap metal. They depict an elderly man sitting on a bench (dimensions: 10 × 10 × 11 cm) and an elderly man carrying the burden of aging (dimensions: 13 × 13 × 20 cm), the latter resembling the Greek mythological Titan Atlas, who was condemned to hold the world on his back for eternity.

ISBN 978-9918-23-184-3

The Elderly

Reflections from Family Practice and Ethics

Professor Pierre Mallia

Kite

Contents

Acknowledgements

The author wishes to thank all the people who contributed to this book and who gave their encouragement. Especially that of President Emeritus George Vella who wrote the foreword and indeed of the continuous support of Professor Godfrey Laferla for his continuous support.

About the author and the project

Professor Pierre Mallia is professor of Family Medicine and Patients' Rights, and a Bioethicist at the Medical School, Mater Dei Hospital, University of Malta. He currently is Chairman of the National Bioethics Consultative Committee and also of the Health Ethics Committee (Research review) of the Department of Health, both within the Ministry of Health and the Elderly.

He is a member of the Committee for Bioethics (CDBIO) of the Council of Europe, and also a former member selected to be on the European Group on Ethics in Science and Technology (EGE) which advised the President of the European Commission.

Locally he teaches Bioethics and Ethics in Science and Technology in several faculties including, Medicine & Surgery, Dentistry, Health Sciences, Science, Engineering, and FEMA. He is also visiting professor at Laennec II University of Lyon where he teaches Research Ethics in the Faculty of Pharmacology.

Following a nine-year stint (with a short interval in between) as President of the Malta College of Family Doctors, he worked to introduce the recognition of Vocational Training for Family Medicine in Malta by the Royal College of General Practitioners (UK). He applied through the University for an Erasmus+ Project (EndCare), on end-of-life in Malta, noticing the lack of both legal clarifications and training on end-of-life care locally. The EndCare project ran for three years which he coordinated and collaborated with the University of L'Aquila in Italy and the Dublin City University, Ireland. There were also professorial participants from England, Ireland, France, Italy, Iran, and from the Pontifical Academy in Rome and UNESCO. Locally the Faculty of Medicine and Surgery collaborated with the Faculties of Laws and that of Theology.

This book is part of the second phase (EndCare2) which has started in 2024 with summer schools, seminars, and conference, plus publication of scholarly papers and books. The local participating faculties has been extended to Health Sciences, Social Wellbeing, and Psychology plus the Malta Health Network, the Hospice Movement, the Malta College of Family Doctors, and the collaboration of the Bioethics Consultative Committee and the Ministry of Health and Elderly. Indeed, their help is invaluable as this project, for the time being will be concentrating on the local scenario. He coordinates the project through the Core Group of representatives from the above-mentioned faculties and organisations and welcomes other organisations who are interested in contributing.

Dedication

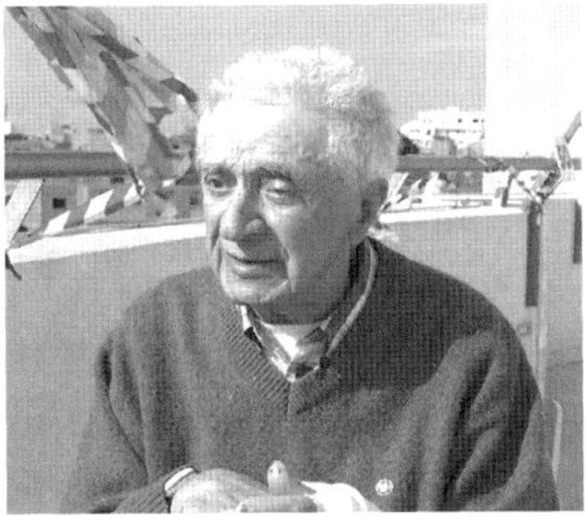

This book is dedicated to Mr Joseph M. Mallia, aged 86, who did a Marathon for Puttinu Cares as an example of Active Aging even under difficult physical disabilities which earned him the Prize for Active Aging of the year 2025. Jospeh passed recently early in 2026.

Joseph M. Mallia was an 86-year-old man who lived at Dar Annunziata, Tarxien. He needed to go into a home as he became progressively blind due to retinal disease and glaucoma also suffered two fractures of the pelvis. Whilst in the home he suffered another fracture of the hip. However, on Christmas Day of 2023, whilst doing physiotherapy he decided to do one thousand paces every day for one year as a marathon in aid of Puttinu Cares foundation.

He organised a team to help him with supervision, accounts and secretarial work and the home gave its permission. He was featured on the front page of *The Sunday Times of Malta* in mid-March 2024 and on several other media shows, including a televised programme to raise funds for the 23 million euro building costs for residences of relatives who go to London for oncological treatment. The feature was a film taken by the crew of *The Sunday Times* which was featured also on Facebook.

Mr Mallia was in the RAF Police and also the Special investigation and Counterintelligence at the time. He then left with his family to work with Ford Moter company whereupon an injury he refused the sum of 2 million dollars (this was over fifty years ago – now equivalent to 50 million) and he was promoted and sent to Ford College to learn on management and 'Time and Space' of mass production.

Back in Malta he helped Janstorp International Malta Ltd. open a textile factory in Kordin and later in Bulebel, and was the Senior Manager under the Swedish General Manager. Following that he went into his dream of furniture industry and eventually employed over 24 workers, but before his last decade before retirement he was called by the then minister for the environment to be an Environment Manager. He is renowned for promoting people by given them training in various subjects and organising a certification ceremony. In this way he motivated and coordinated the cleaning of fields (filled with fridges, oil tanks etc) and re-building rubble walls. The workers respected him as with this certificate they could also work privately. He thus initiated the change in look of what is traditionally mediterranean about our non-urban areas. He was interviewed frequent on television and promoted also the building of Girna on the Island. With a change in government, he continued the same works described here following a chat with the then Minister of the Environment George Vella. President Emeritus George Vella visited him at Dar Annunziata before Mallia passed away on 15 March 2025.

Foreword by President Emeritus George Vella

I am extremely thankful to Professor Pierre Mallia for asking me to write an introduction to his collection of essays entitled "Thinking about the Elderly". This publication is a collection of various articles dealing mostly with end-of-life challenges facing whoever is caring for dying patients, or those who are approaching death.

The range of titles is very vast, and I can safely say that this 'manual' should be compulsory reading for all those who in one way or another deal with end-of-life issues.

This is because the book does not deal only with the theoretical aspects of end-of-life care, but spells out in very great detail, and I would say also in a certain amount of repetition, the steps to be taken in practice by whoever is in charge of dying patients, or patients moving fast towards their death.

This includes carers, nurses, and family doctors, besides hospital staff, depending on where the terminal patient is being cared for.

I highly recommend this book to newly qualified medical doctors, beginning on their careers

This situation is all wrapped up in a quote from Neveloff Dubler, used by Dr Mallia, "In a health care setting, doctrines of justice and patient's rights, translate into concrete decisions based on immediate reality". Decisions have ultimately to be taken by whoever is in charge based on one's knowledge of the subject, one's preparation, and one's clear assessment of the prevailing circumstance of each particular case.

This book provides ample material to inform, but also to whet one's appetite to read further into a subject which as is clearly evident in this book, carries profound medical, moral, religious, ethical, and legal considerations.

The first articles deal with the elderly, the societal roles of grandparents, and their relations with their grandchildren; looking after the elderly at home, cases of abuse, and the increasing vulnerability that comes with age and disease. The 'clinical' problems as well as the 'hotel' problems the elderly face in community homes for the elderly are also looked at.

Chapter 7 is a detailed clinical (semiotics) plan how to examine and look after the aged. Other contributions deal with the risk/benefit an analysis of clinical interventions in the aged, posing questions like 'is it worth treating an elderly patient at that stage of life? Is it in their best interest?' This is logically followed by the consideration between 'ordinary' and 'extraordinary' treatment.

The rest of the chapters go deeper into the subject of end-of-life care and the decisions that have to be taken; pose the question as to how much must one inform the patient; the importance of patient/doctor relationship in palliative terminal care; insisting that doctors need to change from a 'doer to a helper', and from an 'expert problem solver and fixer' to a 'companion'.

Here between the lines, I am seeing a new definition of what 'family medicine' should be all about.

Most of the remaining chapters go into fine detail and discussion on issues such as palliative sedation, and the ethical considerations concerning stoppage of artificial nutrition and hydration when nearing end-of-life. It is repeatedly emphasised that it is not obligatory to take extraordinary measures at end-of-life, and that patients should be allowed to die with dignity.

The subjects discussed deal with issues where science, philosophy, and theology meet. There is also involved biology, technology, ethics, metaphysics and not least spirituality. Such challenging vital end-of-life decisions should be taken within a framework of advanced care planning. One contribution in this book explains on detail a 'consensus statement' to be adopted as guidelines in end-of-life care. It warns against the 'medicalization of death' and stresses the point that we need more discussion on 'end-of-life' in general than on 'euthanasia'. It also debates the fine distinction between 'active killing' as in euthanasia, and 'allowing to die' when death is imminent.

On the same lines there is a most illuminating discussion between what is 'ordinary' treatment, and what can be considered as 'extraordinary treatment', as well as reflections on when CPR should take place, and occasions when it could be in the best interests of the weak fragile patient not to be employed.

The book makes it clear that end-of-life discussions in themselves could form part of palliative care. This takes the reader into the realm of spirituality and the consideration of the patient's morals in reaching end-of-life decisions. The reader will find interesting reflections on Muslim and Christian morals, and their interpretation in actual end-of-life cases.

A concise expression of what is morally and medically acceptable is found in this extract from the Magisterium of the Catholic Church: 'Discontinuing medical procedures that are burdensome, dangerous, extraordinary, or disproportionate to the expected outcome can be legitimate; it is the refusal of 'overzealous' treatment. One is not causing death; one accepts the inability to stop it'.

'Thinking about the Elderly', is anything but bedside reading. It has to be read with utmost attention, and the inevitable repetition, as a matter of fact, help instil important notions and definitions in one's mind.

It is definitely not the last word in care of the elderly, and end-of-life situations. It is however more than just a beginning. The impressive references after each article, show how vast the subject is and how vivid is the ongoing discussion on this aspect of human life. The Erasmus+ EndCare project and the follow up to this EndCare and Active Aging being coordinated by the author continue in this important direction of care.

I definitely recommend this book to whoever is interested in the subject especially carers, medical doctors, psychologists, social workers, and why not, politicians.

Preface

This book is part of the second phase (EndCare2) which has started in 2024 with summer school, seminars, and conference, plus publication of scholarly papers and books. The local participating faculties has been extended to Health Sciences, Social Wellbeing, and Psychology plus the Malta Health Network, the Hospice Movement, the Malta College of Family Doctors, and the collaboration of the Bioethics Consultative Committee and the Ministry of Health and Elderly. Indeed, their help is invaluable as this project, for the time being will be concentrating on the local scenario. I coordinate the project through the Core Group of representatives from the above-mentioned faculties and organisations and welcome other organisation who are interested in contributing.

The book is a collection, or *reader*, of various articles written over several years both in academic journals, books, and the local medica, especial *The Malta Independent on Sunday* on which I have a column, on and off, depending on a busy schedule.[1]

I hope that it will be helpful in helping all of us understand, help and dignify the elderly – a stage in life where many of us will arrive. In this regard it is also about future generations and where we wish to arrive. Any names have been changed and identifable information modified or not mentioned.

Pierre Mallia
Bioethics Research Programme
Medical School, University of Malta

[1] It first appeared as a much shorter version to raise funds for Puttinu Cares through a marathon done by my father (see dedication).

Chapter 1

Does Betty Higden live on? Charles Dickens' contribution to gerontology today[1]

The literature on Dickens's doctors and how Dickens influenced medical knowledge is extensive. He is particularly admired for how he had described disease which were at the time not yet defined, most notably the Fat Boy in *The Posthumous Papers of the Pickwick Club*. However Dickens influenced medicine in many ways. He was concerned about public health, sanitation and housing, and health, illness and disability in general. Not only in his writings, but also in his public life, Dickens was a philanthropist when it came to improving those issues that he wrote about. In particular one notes his being a benefactor to the Children's Hospital of Great Ormond Street, to which he indirectly refers to in his book *Our Mutual Friend*, published only two years after the opening of the hospital. Less reference is made however to his impact on gerontology. In the same book we find the lesser-sung hero Betty Higden, who looks after the child that eventually died in the 'Children's Hospital' and an older boy, Sloppy, who is being given employment by John Harmon.

Saying she does not want to be a burden on Sloppy, who would have to look after her, she decides to leave home and wonder around 'the country' and living on crafts which she is able to do – a strive for financial independence. There is an ensuing debate between Betty and John Harmon, and also with Mrs Boffin, who cares about her well-being and would certainly have provided for her. The fact that Dickens dedicates part of two chapters to this event in Betty's life, or rather, end-of-life, is important and he refers to her at the end of the book in his post script. Here he was referring to the Poor Law, but whereas this

[1] Mallia, P., "Does Betty Higden live on? Dickens's Contribution to Gerontology Today", in *Journal of the International Institute on Ageing*, United Nations, 2014 (4): 23-25.

law applies to all who are poor, why single out an older person? Older people formed an important sub-group in poverty at the time, which today would certainly fall within the realm of gerontology.

If one had to argue that Dickens did not have gerontology in mind, but a simple broader picture of poverty, one would probably be right. But as Chesterton argues in his criticism of *The Old Curiosity Shop*, which again has a reference to an old man who looks after and follows Nell, "the function of criticism, if it has any function at all, can only be one function – that of dealing with the subconscious part of the author's mind which only the critic can express, and not the conscious part of the author's mind, which only the author can express…criticism means saying about the author the very things that would have made him jump out of his boots." Consciously or unconsciously, Betty Higden presents us with a study of gerontology at the time. In *Victorians and Old Age*, Karen Chase argues that Dickens's readers (the broader critics) had another context besides poorhouses in mind, and that was the "reflective reality that aging intensified the vulnerabilities of those already in difficult financial situations".

If space allowed it would be opportune to read slowly through the fourteen pages of Chapter VIII of the Second volume of the Chapman Hall edition which is addressed in its opening to "lords and gentlemen and honourable boards' for the shame at having at their disposal such a law which is misapplied and which people abhor by preferring to die quietly outside in harsh weather "untouched by workhouse hands". For Betty this was "her highest sublunary hope".

As often happens, laws such as the Poor Law, although having an aim (in this case the utilitarian principle of highest possible gain) which is noble, end up causing more harm and pain, not least because of abuse. The Poor Law, for example provided relief to those of low salaries which encouraged farmers to hire people at low salaries knowing they will obtain the difference. But the new Poor Law, intending to curb this abuse, still retained many of the old abuses because it was applied differently from country to county. The new law discouraged people from using the system by turning it quite intentionally into a form of prison with unhealthy food and making it least pleasant as possible.

In gerontology there have been many literary portrayals of aging. Torres says that that criticism in this regard has often focused on them as "a motif, metaphor or symbol of something else: love, time, creativity, memory, mortality". In the postscript referred to earlier he describes his "social experience since Mrs Betty Higden"; Betty being the only character of the whole book that he refers to in the context of the Poor Law, other than the characters which were on the manuscript that he had left behind in the cabin of the infamous train crash when he went to retrieve these characters after assisting many people. He there speaks about two groups of people who supported the Poor-Law relief – one group who would not contend that there were no people who would "prefer death by slow starvation and bitter weather to the mercies of some Relieving Officers and some Union Houses" as was the case for Betty. The other group would contend that there were such people but that there was no reason for what they did. He then refers to *The Lancet*, and newspapers, and common sense which "furnish too abundant evidence against both defenses". Dickens's motif is the Poor Law, but there is a deeper, perhaps unconscious, reading which his readers seemed to have understood.

Perhaps one can question why an old lady should go away when (Sloppy) can look after her. Is that not what many old people do? Even if Dickens lacks proper motive here, he is emphasizing a reality. Betty would have fallen perhaps in the second category of critics he mentioned in the postscript. His portrayal of the Reverend performing the funeral service felt that there was something "not quite right between us and our sister – or say our sister in Law – Poor Law". But Betty wants financial and social independence. Leaving because of Sloppy seems to be the excuse. Like all elderly she does not want to be a burden. But the social system in place does not provide adequate and respectful shelter. Interestingly, just as Betty runs away with funeral money sewn into her dress, so do many elderly people find the same dignity and not wanting to be a burden on their 'Sloppys',put aside money for their own funeral. The psyche of the elderly person has changed little.

Tomalin points out that the *Old Curiosity Shop* has a large number of characters who experience bodily distress or difficulty, attributing these pains as a reminder of Dickens' personal pain – he was suffering from foot pain. Although there may be truth in this, it is speculative. At least Betty's death and her story is as intended as are all his other references to health, poverty and the darker side of London at the time. Notwithstanding the criticism that the novel often received – a criticism which proved unjustified, Chesterton notes that the novel is a return to Dicken's farse of the past. His books had become rather more serious and this was a brilliant return to his former manner. It is also 'vulgar' and written the way English people speak. This includes the title, noticing that no scholar would have used the incorrect title of 'Mutual' friend.

In Betty Higden, Dickens does not only consciously want to work a reprise on the Poor Law satire but perhaps unconsciously (to allow for Chesteron) is telling us something about the way elderly fared. Certainly today it still reveals skeletons in health care systems a when it comes to the study of the elderly. The gerontological lesson Betty continues to teach is not that elderly are too proud to receive (she means to give no 'offence' by her action), "but that I want to be of a piece like, and helpful of myself right through to my death". Old people abhor being a burden but would like the means to maintain dignity.

Betty reminds us of the plight of many elderly people even today who wish to die at home and not be institutionalized, notwithstanding system improvement. As the percentage of elderly people increases, they have become an economic burden! As a physician I find that so many people do not want to end up in an 'old people's home'; we still witness how treatment in these homes is not optimal, for the very reason that they are not hospitals. We witness disappointed relatives thinking that by admitting their loved ones in homes they were going to solve their medical problems as well. Conversely, even if such homes were optimal, there are simply not enough places for everyone. If state homes are not given a pseudo-hospital status, as elderly require medical attention and palliative care almost regularly, would there be an uncanny parallel to keeping the less pleasant in order to encourage the elderly to remain in the community?

On the other hand, if we had to extrapolate and speak about hospitals, how many people are treated in hospitals at the end-of-life, prolonging their life with what they would consider extraordinary care, when at home they would die more peacefully with ordinary measures. We seem to be afraid to allow people to die a normal death and push them into an environment in which they will receive artificial nutrition and hydration. Conversely some die sadly at home because they are not given timely admission into residences for the elderly; they are not too ill to be hospitalized but too ill to be at home anyway. Every country will have to face its own problems with regard to the quality of life of their elderly. But certainly it would be a pity if after all these years we would still find the Betty Higden's who would not avail themselves of the services offered because they are poor in quality and prefer to die alone at home, or, need admission for palliation and cannot receive it. The recent example of the lack of training of the Liverpool Care Pathway, in itself an attempt to give to everyone the palliative care which is given in hospices, can serve as an example– it turned against the system as something which was deliberately removing ANH without the consideration the pathway itself dictated.

The plight of the elderly may often be ignored and Charles Dickens notes the ignorance in their regard: "ladies in carriages would frequently make purchases from her trifling stock, and were usually pleased with her bright eyes and her hopeful speech. In these and her clean dress originated a fable that she was well to do in the world: one might say, for her station, rich.", warning that, "As making a comfortable provision for its subject which costs nobody anything, this class of fable has long been popular." With Europe's elderly population facing poverty, Betty Hidgen reminds us of this plight.

References

Bleakley S. Review of 'The Victorians and Old Age' by Karen Chase, in *Review* 19 www.nbol-19.org. 2009; Available at: http://www.nobol-19.org/view_doc.php?index=54. Accessed September, 2013.

Bosen R. Europe's Elderly Face Poverty. *Journal of the International Institute on Aging* 2013; 23(4):27.

Chesterton GK. *Criticisms and appreciations of the work of Charles Dickens*. London, Vermont.: Everyman's Library; 1992: 52, 210.

Dickens C. *Our Mutual Friend*, Vol. 2. EU: GE Fabbri; 2004: 104.

Kryger M. Charles dickens: Impact on Medicine and Society. *Journal of Clinical Sleep Medicine* 2012; 8(3):333-338.

Newsom R. Poor relief and the new poor law of 1834. In: Schlicke P, editor. *The Oxford Companion to Charles Dickens*. Anniversary Edition ed. Oxford, New York, Auckland, Toronto: Oxford University Press; 2011. p. 464-466, 445.

Tomalin C. Charles Dickens. *A life*. London, New York, Toronto.: Penguin Books; 2012.

Wallace D. Literary Portrayals of Aging. In: Stuart-Hamilton I, editor. *An Introduction to Gerontology*. 1st ed. Cambridge, New York, Melbourne, Madrid: Cambridge University Press; 2011. p. 389-415: 391.

Chapter 2

Young working couples and the elderly; are working parents affecting negatively their mental health[1]

Whilst gender equality is coming of age, the problem of where to leave children during the day remains an elusive one. Whilst childcare centers are encouraged there are considerable doubts (The Guardian, 2009) as to whether leaving children at a very young age in these environments can cause psychological harm or distress both during development and later in life. The alternative in some countries is to leave the children for the day with relatives. In Malta these relatives are usually the parents of one of the spouses, the grandparents of the children themselves.

An article I wrote (Mallia, 2011) was quoted by an economical review that same year (Delia, 2010): "the number of children brought up by relatives is on the rise. This emerging family-support network, while useful for young parents and the economy in general, may be introducing a new cause for tension among the elderly; they want to help their children and at the same time feel they are useful, but if the demands are persistent and overdone – in other words, if they are abused by their children – then the grandparents' support will actually affect their health negatively. It is not in anybody's long term interest that such feature becomes relatively wide-spread."

The size of the island and the tendency for many young couples to live close to their parents fosters a situation where this family-support becomes imperative. The parents of these couples will argue that they feel it is their duty to help as the young couple has a lot of expenses. In this however most are deluded into believing that the young couples cannot take responsibility for their lives. After all, the choice that both

[1] Mallia, P., "Gender issues and the elderly: are working parents affecting negatively the Maltese elderly population?" *United Nations Journal of the International Institute on Ageing*, 2012: 22(2); 2-6.

go to work is an internal family decision which should be carried by them alone in the long run. Certainly gender equality cannot come at the expense of grandparents who have already raised their own children and who are entering or have entered a new phase of life which carries with it more morbidity and perhaps increase the scope of participating less in opportunities for the elderly such as education for the third age.

Factors which may contribute to increased use of the couples' parents include:

1. Close proximity
2. willingness on the part of grandparents
3. Increasing expenses to provide for the new family
4. Avoidance of paying for childcare services and/or disagreement with child care services as a matter of principle
5. If young couples are willing to take their children to childcare centers, some grandparents will prefer to look after them themselves
6. Availability of time of the grandparents to take children to school and to bring them back home and look after them until the parents come to collect them.

Some disadvantages are:

1. Increased stress on elderly (*ibid.*)
2. Fear that if they do not take care of the children, the parents may resort to child care services
3. Lack of time to participate in opportunities for the elderly such as organized daily activities and participating in educational initiatives. (Malta offers the opportunity for education for the 'third age')
4. Children may grow confused as to *where* they can really call home
5. Feelings of guilt if they do not comply
6. Disagreement between the elderly couple on whether they should keep them.

The advantages can be more obvious:

1. Less cost for child care
2. Children are taken care of by parents
3. Less worrying that children are in an institution
4. Elderly may (at least at first) enjoy the opportunity to be with their grandchildren and to be part of their upbringing.

Certainly it can reasonably be argued that whilst one should encourage social participation of the elderly population and taking care of children may be one way to accomplish this, one cannot but be concerned that at this age people are less likely to be able to cope with the demands and stress of taking care of children. Adding to this the legal responsibility which grandparents are taking, of which they may not be aware, one must ask whether this action, if carried too far, constitutes *elderly abuse* and whether social services should be looking into such cases. It is all too easy for working parents to rely unduly on their own parents often one finds that these grandparents look mostly after the children of only one of their siblings. This may point to character problems with the working parents who may have been more demanding when young and continue to be so when adults.

To understand the individual stress grandparents go through and the denial some may experience one has to look into the narrative of cases. Two such cases are briefly viewed here. The names and some details relating to the case are altered for privacy purposes.

Case 1

The Farrugias are an elderly couple who have three married children. All of their children are married to partners who work as well. One of their daughters brings her two girls very early in the morning so that her father can walk the children to school. Later during the day he picks them up from school and the children stay at their grandparents until they are picked up by either their mother or their father at around 7pm.

The grandfather discusses this problem with the general practitioner. His wife is very depressed and he suspects that the stress of the situation contributes to her depression. He is a very calm man but also complains that his daughter and her husband 'abuse' because 'even in summer they do not give him a break'. Since they still have to work in summer they send their children to summer school and he still has to take them and pick them up 'in the heat of the afternoon'. He complains that the only time he is unengaged is when his daughter goes on holiday with her family for one or two weeks in summer. He is also concerned that he is not appreciated: 'Lanqas grazzi ma jgħidulhek' (they don't even thank you).

He says that were it not for the children he would like to go 'to one of those university courses they offer'.

Case 2

Mr and Mrs Grech are an elderly couples who often call their general practitioner when their grandchildren are sick. The general practitioner notices that every time he sees the children the parents are never around. The elderly couple explain that their daughter is married to a foreigner who had trouble finding a job; they stay with the two boys during the day and when they are sick they come to the flat of their daughter so that they are not taken out. The flat is four storeys high and they both complain, when noticing that the general practitioner takes time to catch his breath, that they too feel they are unable to cope with those stairs but that they do it or their daughter.

Slowly the general practitioner gets to know the family more and finds out that their other daughter is also a working mother but takes full responsibility for her own children. They say that the mother of these children was always a little more difficult.

One day the general practitioner is called, but this time asked to visit them at their own house. During the house-call they explain that their daughter has argued with her husband as he wanted to buy an expensive Mercedes and she disagreed as they were still paying for the flat. She left him and went to live with her parents. The situation lasted several months until they finally got back together again. During this time the daughter's husband visits his family regularly and relations are quite stable whilst they talk things out.

One day her father complains with the general practitioner about the stressfulness of the situation and how his wife tends to cope worse. When the general practitioner asks why they do not explain to their daughter that they should tone down their commitment he says that 'they have expenses'. The general practitioner explains that he has four children and that he does not abuse his parents or that of his working wife. They try to manage. The father responds by saying, yes 'but you are a doctor'; implying that as a doctor he has more income. Frustrated at this comment the doctor politely points out that he drives a small Toyota and has not yet bought a Mercedes after all these years in practice! He explains that perhaps by their help they are actually allowing them to carry out caprices which, had they been in charge of their children, they may not have done.

Both cases illustrate errors in judgement of all parties concerned. What both cases have in common is that only one of the siblings makes use of the parents to look after her children and this may be something worthwhile studying further. In the first case the father shows concern for his wife and the lack of consideration of his daughter. He complains that he is not appreciated. His error lies in not being able to say 'no' and to fall under the pressure of the circumstance. Even if he can look after the children during the normal scholastic terms, he can say no to summer – he is not understanding that working mothers do not have summer off and must still work. The mother on her part does not consider that in agreeing to look after her children during the school months, this does not include summer holidays. If not an error in judgement it is certainly an abusive situation which both yield to in their own way, perhaps giving an explanation.

In the second scenario the father clearly gives himself an excuse that his daughter and her husband have financial problems. Rather than allowing them to learn from the over-expense of the car, he gives in to the situation once the tension in the marriage has been resolved and perhaps not to feel he is the cause should the marriage fail. In this he convinces himself that they have financial problems, when in reality they are non-existence in so far as all couples experience financial difficulties in the first years of marriage and must learn from their mistakes. The daughter indulges happily in the support the family provides and takes everything for granted. Rather than complaining to her husband that he should not have bought the car whilst her parents are looking after their children, the only excuse she gives is the fact that she would have preferred the money to go into continuing to pay for the flat. Not only does she not acknowledge the sacrifice of her parents, but she now moves into their home leaving her husband alone in the flat. Rather than dealing with the issue as a family she decides to threaten to leave by actually moving out; yet she allows him to 'live' with them during the day when he is not at work, at her parent's house.

Such cases can merit further individual analysis and this brief analysis may indeed not be complete. Suffice to say that statistical studies may not be enough to illustrate the problem and qualitative analysis of the problem is merited. Certainly the issue is related to gender issues relating to work. This newly social construct cannot be challenged by retrogressive steps – pushing women back into homes. Neither however should guilt feelings be forced upon women who choose not to work because of their family.

There are possible solutions to the problem. This first is acknowledging the situation exists. Following several articles in the media no one seems to have acknowledged the problem. We tend as a society to wait not only for empirical evidence but perhaps also for a certain amount of harm to occur before one takes political action. Certainly in similar situations the precautionary principle advocated by UNESCO has not resulted in much (Ten Have, 2006).

Some solutions may be:

1. Monitoring by social services the well-being of elderly people looking after children, including keeping good statistics and evaluations of impact.
2. Making use of family doctors to detect the families concerned and identify any problems.
3. Re-thinking issue of gender – that equality is not necessarily sameness and that the way we look at work may have to be different in order not to have a negative impact on the family.
4. Acknowledge that childcare centers, although practical for many are not a solution for all and that children being exposed more than a maximum amount of hours per week to such centers may constitute abuse and abandonment. Certainly if parents work 40-hour weeks, one needs to include times traveling to and from work which means that children may be spending up to 50 hours or more, if overtime is included.
5. Not looking at the problem in an isolated way but identifying other social phenomena, such as the rise in teenage single motherhood, which may be related to the problem. These young girls, for example, may be viewing married life negatively; even though they themselves may be the cause of much anxiety and work to their own (elderly) parents.

The use of the word 'elderly' has been used liberally throughout this article, which may indeed be a limit to its arguments. Thus newly retired adults may be quite energetic to take care of their grandchildren and the problem only seems to surface as they start getting older. No distinction has been made between the young-old and the old-old. In fact the problem probably pertain more to the young-old. Nevertheless studies and observations from general practice will show whether there is an increased in morbidity, as is being advocated here, in this population in countries where family ties remain very closely knit.

In a society which is trying to avoid ageism and where the usefulness of the elderly population is encouraged, one has to beware that usefulness is in itself a misnomer. One thing is feeling useful; it is quite another to 'use' someone because of their life status. This can be seen as 'ab'use. Adler has often pointed out that elderly should not feel inadequate and their worth comes from what they have accomplished in life and not from what they accomplish now. It is this that needs merit and certainly accomplishing a family and having grandchildren should not bring with it a necessity to look after grandchildren more than their parents do for them not to feel inadequate.

It was once argued, something which still holds true for many families, that in trying to prove they are still alive, elderly pamper their grandchildren as they seems to be the only ones to take notice of them (Way, 1956). In this they interfere with their education by the very nature of spoiling. How this affects children of working parents leave many unanswered questions. Are children identifying more with the authority of grandparents? Are grandparents replacing (and can they) the role of the parents? Are children, on the other hand, continuing to be spoilt all the time – after all the grandparents are not the parents? Certainly in recognizing the stressfulness which is hitting this section of the elderly population we may only be touching the tip of the iceberg. The subjects are also the children. It would be interesting how this subject can be made to work in view of the call for solidarity between generations made by Archbishop Paul Cremona (Cremona, 2012); sticking the right balance that elderly continue to play a role in our society which does not impinge on their health should be our goal.

References

Cremona, P. (2012). *Solidarjetà bejn il-ġenerazzjonijiet (Solidarity amongst generations)*. Flimkien, January 2012. p. 4.

Delia, E. P. (2010). *Catholic social teaching, economic thought and four hundred thousand Maltese*. Malta: APS Bank Publications.

Mallia, P. (2011). *Articles in clinical ethics*. Malta: Bioethics Research Programme, University of Malta.

The Guardian. (2009). *Working mothers have unhealthy children*, on guardian.co.uk, Tuesday 29 September.

Ten Have, H. (2006). The activities of UNESCO in the area of ethics. *Kennedy Inst Ethics J, 16*, 333-351.

Way, L. (1956). *Alfred Adler. an introduction to his psychology.* USA; Canada; Australia: Pellican books.

Chapter 3
Elderly abuse[1]

Recently a conference was organized on elderly abuse. I was rather disturbed by the ethical input as the concept is certainly not merely a philosophical one and is very elusive. Certainly it is easy to speak about the responsibility of doctors to report such cases, but when it comes to family medicine, the problem is not so simple as I hope to show with the following cases from my own experiences – cases which I have been using with consultant geriatricians in the teaching of ethics in the elderly population.

In the first case a patient visited my clinic and expressed concern at how her aunt was being treated. Her aunt, a spinster, had invited her nephew years before to live with her, when he got married. Of course years go by and children come – in this case two boys – and the children grow old and demand their own room. What initially is pocket money to buy sweets starts becoming some sort of obligatory salary and instead of the family paying any rent, out of the generosity of this women, the wife demanded some compensation for washing of the clothes and shopping. As the boys required a room of their own, this now elderly lady sleeps under the stairs. Were it not for the stairs not having a board making it into a cupboard, it was much like Harry Potter.

The abuse escalated over the years. The boys would verbally and physically abuse the woman if she did not give them money. The mother would take the rest. The lady slowly became very depressed and her only outlet out of the house was a visit to this patient of mine who was now in front of me. She said that she never knew about the whole story as of course the woman was afraid to speak and to be thrown out of her own house. The solution initially was to bring this

[1] Published in *The Malta Independent on Sunday*, 8 September 2010.

woman for a consultation with a consultant geriatrician. The story was confirmed, and social services arranged for immediate transfer into an old people's home for her safety. The tragedy of course was that the abusive family were in the end the people who gained the most. They now automatically had the house to themselves and it seemed that even legally there was nothing one can do. The lady would not sign any contract as she did not want to create scenes.

In a second case an elderly lady was abused by her single daughter who lived with her. She spoke to her sisters (the daughter's aunts) who sided somewhat with the daughter, who used to speak like a martyr that she could not get married because of her mother. One day the elderly lady was admitted to hospital with bruises, which the daughter claimed were due to a fall. A long-standing story of physical abuse transpired from what the mother related in hospital. The story was very traumatic to the mother as she tried even to play it down. Relatives however confirmed that the daughter had often said that she had to use violence. It was a very difficult and painful period for all and in the end, following considerable threats by the daughter of 'malafama', the woman was taken to a home. Again the old lady felt that she did not deserve this treatment – being kicked out of her home. Often she was on the verge of returning upon conviction and feigned repentance of the daughter.

In a third case a woman with five sons and a daughter presented with confusion and dementia. She lived with the daughter and was depressed because one of her sons, who was at loggerheads with the husband of the daughter, would not visit her in her daughter's house. He would not put aside the feud for his mother and being the elderly and dominant brother demanded that the rest accept that the mother be put into a home so that all could see her whenever they wanted to. This was a nice family all in all but they could not resolve this issue until one day I had to admit the mother to hospital for chest pain. When she recovered no one would take responsibility and she was (abusively) left in hospital. A couple of weeks later the woman was transferred to a home where she died a month later.

All three cases have considerable psychological baggage. In the first case we see outright abuse which escalates over time. The people themselves are not bad people and in fact think they are doing a service to this old lady. The wife buys her food, cooks her the diet she prefers, does her washing, and sees to her needs. The boys have got used to pocket some money and become violent by pushing and sneering if she does not give them what they request. But boys are young and correction by the mother is to no avail. They grew up in an environment in which no particular respect was given to this lady. What about the family doctor? What about him? He is never brought in unless really needed and in this case it is the family doctor and not her former doctor who is called. They were ironically trying to arrange to get her into a home. They succeeded without any effort as it were. The wife was the first to go and take back the television set when the woman died in the home a few years later.

The morale of the story is that we should listen to relatives who complain and try to set up a meeting. Now this is not always easy as we do not know whether this niece was simply envious. I knew her for some time and knew her character well. But in family medicine you learn and continue to learn. Things are not always what they seem. It was very clear-cut however in this case and we could take the immediate necessary action. Malta being Malta the family were simply told that the woman had to be admitted to a home because of her age. No action was taken and no evidence was gathered.

The second case presents a very painful picture. Of course not all the details can be given. People taking care of elderly are not always competent to do so. They often have problems of their own. They find it difficult to run a social life unless they have the confidence to leave the 'patient' at home alone. Pressure by the patient often accumulates over years were the person feels guilty even to go out. It starts with some verbal abuse and then some pushing and forceful shifting when cleaning them and anger when they trip or soil their clothes. Then, if they do not eat what they prepare, perhaps some forceful feeding and even a hit here and there. Suddenly it escalates to pushing and hitting. The person feels guilty and buys gifts, whitewashes the bedroom and is all caring for a while – until the tension rises again. This cycle is well documented in domestic violence. The downside is that it rarely can be detected, even by family doctors, unless the person speaks out. If there is dementia it becomes more difficult to prove.

The situation is usually detected by an element of suspicion. In this case recurrent falls were the excuse for the bruises but whenever these occur the doctor was never called in. It is often also the case that another member of the family speaks to his or her own doctor about the situation. A family conference often reveals a considerable amount of information. Of course the brothers and sisters of the women were all in sympathy for the daughter as their sister was described as always being somewhat of a fuss-pot. But when confronted with whether they wished their sister to continue to live in those conditions they finally gave in. All the evidence was there. It was merely explained to the daughter that over time she developed a severe amount of tension and she was venting out her frustrations on her mother. In this case even the gifts were related to periods when the daughter had expressed her attitude to her aunts.

Taking action is not easy. It is not easy to take an elderly person out of the home. And often the aggressor is simply suffering from a depression and is not getting any help. They feel let down that after years of taking care of parents or relatives, they are then seen as the aggressors. Perhaps leaving things alone as we do in Malta helps. However it certainly does not help as a deterrent. We should heed people when they tell us that they cannot cope with the elderly they take care of any longer. Often taking care of elderly has its benefits monetarily which can be the cause of people *not* seeking help, as in this case. The paid-for electricity and water bills come in handy. The situation is complicated. But there are two things which can be readily done.

The first is to recognise family medicine as a speciality and train this specialist in the detection of any form of domestic violence and equip them with the tools of what to do and when to intervene. It is a pity that the attachment with practices in the current vocational trainee system is not enough to get sufficient exposure. It is also a pity that doctors are still being sent out into the community without vocational training, unless, that is, they want to work in health centres, where the EU directive only seems to be interpreted to apply. Family medicine is not a speciality just for the sake of being called a speciality. In many countries where vocational training is in place, the trainee doctor spends three years working in a practice. They learn from colleagues, have discussions and learn that the solution can be handled in the community. Often it is unfortunate that locally we have to wait until the patient is admitted to hospital for some reason.

The second is to continue investing in homes in the community. Ideally these homes should be in villages and give preference to the villagers so that they can be close to relatives and relatives close to them. The paradoxical problem is that we have put too many restraints and conditions to have homes. Recently relatives of mine inherited a large house and I had the idea of starting a home for the elderly. The limiting factor were the new regulations. At the time there was a different parliamentary secretary for the elderly with whom I could speak quite frankly. When she gave me the lists of conditions, including having not more than two people in a room (and soon it was to be one) and private toilets and special beds etc., etc., one could realise that things are laid down in good faith, but the reality is that there are many people living in home – especially homes runs by nuns, where these conditions are not met. And they work very well and people are happy. To set conditions is easy; you may not realise you are blocking progress.

This is happening across the board and is a sign of progress. A patient of mine who owns a restaurant and wants to have another floor upstairs has paid over a hundred thousand euros in permits and conditions and it was even imposed upon him that he should have a parking lot and a ramp for wheel chairs. Now if this was a new venture, perhaps it could have been justified. But all he wanted to do was create a pizzeria upstairs. Business is impeded in this way. It is the same with those who wish to offer a service for the elderly. It is true that profits are made, but the fees are already prohibitive as they are. People pay up to one hundred euros per day in a private home at present. But if the investment is prohibitively high the results are that either people are not able to afford (except the rich – as it is today), or that investors are simply discouraged.

The solution is that if government wants conditions, perhaps it can help in some way. The alternative of having large contractors building large old-peoples' homes is simply having other large SVPRs. Rather than considering large home as the Żejtun or Bormla home, we should consider the large houses which can be converted easily into small home which can accommodate twenty or so residents in their own village. After all, we boast lateral thinking as a national pride.

Chapter 4
The vulnerability of elderly

A case

Mrs A was a 75-year-old elderly person admitted to emergency care with dehydration and hypoglycaemia. She said that since she moved slowly her daughter had begun to push her to move faster and that the wounds had come from falls during these occasions in which she hit object – which is what she would report to the general practitioner. Later she claimed that the daughter hit her when she would not eat. The most recent was an injury to her forehead which she claimed was due to a recent push when she hit the corner of the table. She said that on one occasion, when she did not like the food her daughter had prepared, the latter had splashed the plate onto her face.

The general practitioner had noticed in the past some signs of possible abuse which were always denied. S, noticing that the doctor had become suspicious started to call in another general practitioner who complied with the reasons the daughter used to give him. S had a personality disorder, had broken up with a boyfriend with whom she would often fight. There was a long history when the first general practitioner was always called after hours by S because her mother had fainted. Invariably these were found to be hysterical attacks feigning unconsciousness. She would revive when the general practitioner said in front of Mrs A that he wanted to send her to hospital for loss of consciousness. Her blood glucose was always good on these occasions. It always transpired that the daughter had made a scene. One day the former general practitioner was called because of the above episode who took the opportunity to send her to hospital. He called the hospital to ask the casualty officers to inquire about any abuse.

The mother had finally given in to the above history when at casualty and was kept in hospital. It was then arranged that due to the abuse she was to be transferred into a home. The daughter denied any abuse saying that her mother was confused and that she had dementia. This did not prove clinically to be the case. Mrs A insisted that no one tell her daughter what she had said about her as she did not want to bring her into trouble.

After two years in the home Mrs A died. S continued to complain that they had taken her mother away from her and that the nursing home nurses had killed her. The general practitioner visited Mrs S three to four times a year and on these occasions Mrs A would always burst out crying complaining about her fate to end up in a home. "I did not deserve to end up like this, but I could not continue living with my daughter. She is repentant now, you know, but I cannot trust her". These and similar remarks always confirming the abuse were made to the doctor and nurses many times.

Background philosophy

The above case reveals how human rights can be violated in circumstances which may be very difficult to prove. Home carers may even with good intention not be competent to look after their elderly relatives. It can frequently happen that sons or daughters who remain at home may have issues and some form of personality traits which certainly would not make them fit to look after their parents. In this regard general practitioners can do a lot of work to detect suspected abuse. But in a country where patient registration is not in place, the carer may easily bring in another doctor fresh to the family who may comply with the reasons given for the injury. This does not help in collecting evidence to build up a case which can be used to protect the vulnerable person.

Human rights and anthropological reflection

In his book *Vulnerability – Challenging Global Perspectives*, Henk Ten Have, former Chief of the UNESCO Section on Ethics, gives a detailed analysis, probably the first of its kind, on vulnerability in all its facets. Much of what is described is applied also to elderly. In order to understand the context of such cases as the above, one need realise that the carers may not be wholly responsible, especially in countries that encourage people to keep elderly at home or in their environment. Of course these carers have little training and can easily come to suffer from frustration, burn out and anger due to lack of support. This does not justify violence, but it does justify the need for support networks even when being taken care of by family members or friends, in order to persuade these people for their need for help both personally and socially (Ten Have, 2017).

From an anthropological perspective Ten Have argues that vulnerability is universal, passive, and positive (Ten Have, 2017, p. 109). It is universal because vulnerability is a shared human condition; we are all subject to vulnerability. An accident may make us vulnerable. Being vulnerable has various universal dimensions – it may be in the body, in personal existence, in relationships and in dependencies. Elderly are subject to all of these, perhaps especially in the body and in many instances, dependency. Relationships can also be affected because of ageism. We are also vulnerable because of the existential nature of being older; which means not being able to do things as efficiently and as effectively as before. Ten Have asserts that, "the possibility of stereotyping or discriminating is eliminated if (this) anthropological vulnerability is recognised". Awareness that everyone can be vulnerable is important for professional relationships in healthcare. Although this may sound utilitarian, it is also a driving force for a principled-approach. Ten Have quotes Emanuel Levinas who saw vulnerability as a breakdown of autonomy. Human beings are passive in many ways. They have no control over becoming older, with all the implications. It signifies the collapse of the idea of self-mastery in many respects. Ten Have puts emphasis on the title of his book – that of challenging bioethics – in bioethicists' contemporary discourse. In research ethics, for example, the older research subject is seen as possessing the characteristics of being "well-informed, rational, competent, (and) self-determining". The anthropological perspective shifts the emphasis therefore from agency to susceptibility and passivity. Quoting Jacques Derrida, Ten Have notes that that there is a non-power rather than a power (which seems to be the emphasis of empowered patients in bioethics).

This idea of anthropological vulnerability can enable us towards the third condition (after universal and passive) – that of positivity.

Anthropology enables us towards a more positive interpretation of vulnerability. Since it is a fundamental human condition, one cannot oppose vulnerability and autonomy. It comes a priori to being autonomous, in fact, and therefore should be recognised as a quality all humans can have as autonomous beings. Ten Have therefore argues that vulnerability should be an ethical principle, which ought to be reflected as a principle of protection or respect for the vulnerable. This translates into a duty to prevent harm from occurring to people. The UNESCO Universal Declaration on Bioethics and Human Rights presents the principle of respect for the vulnerable. The implication is that it is an acknowledged human condition and does not necessarily mean it is bad or negative. "Respect however does not mean acceptance, resignation, or denial". Being a shared feature of the human species it forces upon us, from a political perspective, a reorientation from a focus on ourselves to the needs of the other.

Another anthropological reflection is given by Harri Englund in his discourse on 'moral panics' (Englund, 2009). By moral panics (in academic usage) one means an extraordinary collective action that seeks to counter perceived threats to fundamental values. Englund relates the public's perception on corrupt practices in various countries which led to moral panic and hence to a 'Mob Justice'. Although a mob panic in the case of elderly abuse may not be the case, it is certainly publicly perceived enough in Malta to have led to media coverage and academic reflection and certainly brings many patients to general practitioners complaining about siblings, relatives, neighbours or even carer who abuse elderly. The response fortunately is timely and as described has been addressed to a certain extent within the law with the intention of following up on the issue. Certainly financial abuse has been widespread and perhaps has been the result that many old people used to leave property and money to ecclesiastical authorities after being asked to do so for indulgencies. This led to many people who volunteer to 'look after' older people and gain their trust, only to coerce them into leaving their property in their will to them after convincing them that they are the only people who actually care about them. When it comes to violence this is perhaps more covered up and less known.

Interestingly, Carolyn Fluehr-Lobban (2015), has asserted that ethics should be in the interest of anthropologists so as not to be side viewers but to be in a position to effect positive change. She quotes the American Anthropological Association's Code of Ethics that "anthropologists may choose to move beyond disseminating research results to a position of advocacy, but making this choice is not an ethical responsibility", admitting that advocacy is of course subject to an anthropologists point of view. She affirms nevertheless that "ethics, and by extension, morality, is central to our work, our discipline, and our legitimacy as a profession". Whilst both the anthropology of ethics is fundamental to anthropology, acting as 'advocates' upon the findings may decrease the credibility of research as it may poise the anthropologist as biased. In other words, the anthropologist ceases to rest in research equipoise. This may be counterproductive as often advocates do quote research as part of their biased political agenda and if such research is put in doubt and especially if its repeatability and methods are put into question, then anthropology would lose its credibility. In doing anthropological work on ethics, therefore, one must be equipoised unless one is to be perceived as trying to push forward a particular a priori point of view. Although total equipoise may not be possible in real terms, once it is made clear that anthropologists themselves will advocate action on outcomes, the standard is further put into question. Rather the anthropologist must concentrate on the repeatability of work and indeed cherish an equipoise that in itself will be useful ethically to make the results of her work useful.

The anthropological foundation of care can be seen from ancient times. Gabriella Gambino points out the Latin philological-literary tradition which give two meanings to care. One, which can be seen in Horace and Virgil, reflects stress and anxiety; the other being more about virtues – solicitous, thoughtful, conscientious, co-participatory, – a meaning reflected in Seneca (Gambino, 2017). She notes that even Heidegger has noted that care is seen as having significance in phenomenology as 'taking care of' and 'having concern'. Heidegger has been elaborated in his ethical significance of 'care' both in the doctor-patient relationship and within the concept of Justice and explained through the meaning of 'being-with' as a consequence of 'being-in-the-world', and 'being-thrown' in the situation of *Dasein* (mankind) (Mallia, 2014).

Principle of justice

A big responsibility of political philosophy is social justice. Ten Have argues for a broader perspective of the concept of justice in order to realise the scope of social justice while recognising the need to accept vulnerability as a human condition and not as something which is simply an unfortunate occurrence for a few. He notes the connection between human rights and vulnerability. Human rights are a direct result of the anthropological vulnerable condition of humans. Historically humans have been subject to slavery and other conditions. It is a vulnerability which either the environment or other humans can impose on humanity. However human rights should not only provide general protection but, he argues, should be directed to special vulnerabilities through "decreasing social inequalities and safeguarding socio-cultural conditions for human flourishing". Once the vulnerability of the elderly is seen through an anthropological lens the reading of Human Rights declarations becomes broadened into a general principle of respecting the vulnerability of humans in their general ontological condition. That of aging is a natural condition which may lead to inequalities and decreasing the flourishing of humans who age. Whilst a lot has been done to increasing the scope of aging, the vulnerability of elderly living in society can still be perceived, even from the over-powering of those who look after them. Vulnerability explains the *emergence* of human rights and as such the emergence of the rights of elderly should be a sine qua non. This has been recognised by UNESCO and the World Health Organisation. The scope of human rights inspires ethical and normative actions which go beyond law-making. It should not focus mainly on the individual but on human nature as a collective ideal to protect the species. One recalls how Bronovski in his book and Television series *The Ascent of Man* describe an elderly person who is part of a nomadic group still existent at the time, who sits down and awaits his death once he felt that he cannot continue to journey with the group. Civilisation would not have been possible if humans remained nomadic. The fact that they stopped moving meant they could build dwellings and structures – and elderly continued to live in these societies. They were not a burden even in nomadic groups but simply could not (as a personal decision) keep up with the group which moved with the season. Looking after the elderly was a further natural development with buildings and civilisation. It has become more evident today due to increasing life expectancy and since families now do not remain in their homes and move to other cities. Working parents can also have an impact on leaving someone at home alone. Elderly therefore have stopped dwelling in the same place where their children have grown and married and continued to build their families. It is interesting that Atul Gawande, in his now classic book *Being Mortal*, notes that where this still occurred until some time ago, as in Indian communities, the elderly continued to be the leaders and owners of the land (Gawande, 2015).

Ten Have goes on to say that the relationship between human rights and bioethics is worrisome, quoting Richard Ashcroft who sees bioethical discourse as 'less threatening' than that of human rights (*ibid*, Have, 2017), implying that speaking about morality alone is not as effective. For example, although many bioethicists see themselves as being clinical ethicists for the simple reason that they are capable of giving advice to clinicians, this does not translate into a social movement to effect change. End-of-life issues, including the elderly by default, goes beyond theoretical applied philosophy and requires a being-with the patient. Just as doctors cannot train to become doctors only through theory found in books but must learn to examine patients in their bio-psycho-social context, it is the same to do proper ethics. Clinical ethics is incorporated into the clinical triad of taking a good history, doing a proper examination and ordering tests, which all give meaning and input into ethical outcome. This is the reason why, after decades of moral guidelines for end-of-life, health care professional still find difficulty in applying them in real life. The Erasmus+ EndCare project (2016) attempts to address these issues. Many texts (Gawande, 2015; Nutik Zitter, 2017; O'Mahony, 2016)) reflect how health professionals complain about the way we die now. Even cardiopulmonary resuscitation has been described as 'flogging of dead horses' in many situations. It is done because there is a procedure and the vulnerability of an elderly man may not be recognised as a condition in which CPR ought not to be given because of the harm it will do. Rather we need to ask whether we are treating the person (the patient) or the family (who wish to see that all has been done), or indeed to protect ourselves from litigation.

Certainly, a deeper exploration between bioethics and human rights is needed, the former reducing the notion of vulnerability as a 'failed autonomy' (Ten Have, 2017, p. 172). Human rights have also been criticised as being about individual rights rather than about those who have the power to change structures. It is not only about distribution of resources, but rather about the power over the distribution of resources. This has deep implications for doing bioethics, which should concern itself for injustice, inequalities and the balance of power. When applied to the elderly we see a change in all three of these three conditions. We are aware that an injustice is being done on an elderly person who is being given futile CPR. It is often done merely for medico-legal purposes, or because someone else has taken over the 'power' of attorney. Seeing vulnerability as a human condition may make us reflect deeper on the significant difference between providing CPR to someone who may benefit and someone who will only be harmed to wake up in more pain and discomfort from fractured ribs. The purpose of giving back life has been somewhat lost. What life is being given back to someone who is dying only to wait for another episode of resuscitation to be repeated?

Justice also requires us to recognise vulnerability as a human condition and to actively focus our action on it. Being vulnerable means being in a weak position; and being unable to secure a fair share of benefits. The vulnerable become dependent and the power shifts to the person who is in their charge. Being vulnerable means losing the power to protect oneself and indeed living in an oppressed state. For this reason older people may have to be removed from their homes simply to protect them from someone who knowingly or unwittingly is causing them harm or abusing them as the case above describes. Vulnerability has to be reduced by remedying structures that produce this vulnerability. It is all well and good to encourage people to keep the elderly in the community and to encourage families to keep them by providing salaries, but a framework or support for the carer and vigilance are also necessary. Training should probably also be provided. Ten Have introduces a framework of *Obligations, Responsibilities, Institution-building, and Representation* (Ten Have, 2017 pp. 177-178). Whilst he argues for this on a global perspective, it is reasonable to start on a local level as well. We need to define what the obligations of the carer and the state are. If we are introducing a support network of people, their obligations have to be defined. What are the responsibilities of the carer and the structures? If harm is imposed, then a system of recognising negligence has to be in place. But negligence, by definition requires that people know what their duty of care is. A carer must know what under the law is considered abuse. Support networks have to be able to recognise the need for change to prevent harm. If the carer is not performing due diligence then the support he or she is receiving must be stopped and alternatives considered for the elder person.

Capabilities approach

Ten Have presents the 'capabilities approach' which was advocated by Michael Higgins, the President of Ireland, when he stated a basic question to call for a change in social consciousness which paces human flourishing at the centre of political action. He asked, 'what kinds of human capabilities do particular societies value, encourage, genuinely enable, or block?'[1]. He notes that well-being and human flourishing are not the same as income, satisfaction, or happiness. Development therefore means expanding human capabilities and not more economic income. This is indeed conducive to a quest for meaning. Central to the argument of the model is therefore not focussing on commodities but how to convert commodities into achievements. Ten Have notes that an important advantage of this approach is that it regards older people as resourceful persons who contribute to their families and society, rather than being passive and dependent or vulnerable. This applies also to disabled people. There is no mention, he notes, of vulnerable populations in the capabilities approach, but further down he points out that the implications for this approach is that in order to sustain the capabilities of disabled (and older) persons there is a need for a new approach for social cooperation and not only instituting 'atypical' social arrangements such as custodial care and redesigning of public places.

Therefore, although it is not immediately apparent how vulnerability can be understood within the perspective of the capabilities approach, Ten Have offers several arguments. First there is the concept of

[1] Ten Have, op. Ct., pp179-188.

vulnerability as a limitation of capabilities. Vulnerability, as had been argued, should be regarded as an anthropological and characteristic of human beings. Quoting Nausbaum he reflects that human capabilities are the basic powers for freedom as they are the power to do something. Regarding vulnerability as a limitation of capabilities allows therefore for a conceptual shift – that "the main divergence is in the opportunity to do or to be". "For vulnerable persons opportunities are constrained either because of individual characteristics or due to social, economic, and physical conditions". The development of appropriate environments is therefore a necessity. The difficulty of course is that, he points out that capabilities are not isolated items but that there may be several interconnected multiple capabilities which are affected. He observes that one interpretation of "vulnerability as capability constraint opens up specific remediation possibilities in order to enhance, expand, or recover capabilities". He concludes that the advantage of a capabilities approach is that is accepts vulnerability as a human condition and that vulnerable people are therefore not victims or passive recipients of protection but that they should be enabled to develop their capabilities and capacities. It is about what they are able to do.

Ten Have also notes challenges for this approach. The central aim should be the achievement of well-being, but the approach is confronted with practical challenges. Although it has had an "enormous global impact on social policy, economics, and development studies" it is not clear how legal and political structure can be created that secure a minimum level of central capabilities. Health justice, for example, implies more than just health policies. It is important to reinforce the social context that is required for being healthy – the challenge being to address the material and social constraints to be healthy.

It has been argued that the challenge of justice in health care is to see it as a manifestation of the phenomenon of beneficence (Mallia, 2012). The principles of biomedical ethics are in fact manifestations of the principle which is in fact the phenomenon of the health care profession – patient encounter – beneficence. 'Being-in-the-world' is a human condition and 'being-thrown-into-the-world' is a factor that makes us vulnerable. The authenticity of the doctor-patient relationship comes from a subjective shift to recognising 'justice as care', with care being interpreted in the Heideggerian phenomenology of 'concern'. The very fact of concern as a state of mankind signifies the anthropological and evolutionary importance of vulnerability as a human condition which implicitly shows us as 'being-as' – that is, it is a normal state of human nature and 'being' as potentially vulnerable. This inherently required communities to address in order to survive and help one another survive.

Dynamic of vulnerability

Vulnerability arises when older people show physical and/or mental degeneration that cannot be addressed entirely (Gambino, 2017). For older people Dyer and Ostwald (2011) argue that there is a balance between the physical and mental competence and the environment of the individual. The environment is broadly interpreted by them according to a model which refers to any external demands on the individual. These demands can come from lack of social support, unsafe environments, poverty which leads to lack of necessities or inaccessible health care. The personal competence is affected by resilience, health status, life-style, ability to manage activities of daily living, and the management of chronic illness. It is interesting that all of these factors make the individual prone to abuse.

Robert Gordon and Deborrah Brill (2001) note that family situations were not the only places where abuse and neglect of the elderly were discovered. Nursing homes and other long-term institutions were also identified where frail, elderly people were vulnerable to mistreatment. Questionable management added to the growing evidence that not all was well into a growing area of care in which, as in Malta, there was also a growing private industry involved. They explain abuse under several categories based on their research:

- *The stressed caregiver hypothesis*, in which the foremost explanation was the stress that the caregiver was undergoing led to both physical and emotional abuse of the elderly and that this was thus a consequence of overworked and under-appreciated family caregivers, usually women, who had responsibility for the elderly.
- *The learned violence hypothesis*, where the family carers are brought up from childhood in an environment where violence was used.

This could even have been spouse violence. The Caregiver thus 'learns' to be violent and this is exposed only later when the situation comes into contact with the health services. The care giver could have been the victim of child abuse or spouse abuse by the person he or she is taking care of.

- *The psychopathic hypothesis* describes researcher's findings that various pathologies from substance abuse to personality disorder and psychiatric conditions were found among those responsible for abuse.
- *The dependency hypothesis*, finally, is a little more complicated and focuses on both victim dependency and caregiver dependency. In the latter the research focuses on the extent to which the mental and physical incapability leads to dependency and consequently dependence upon a caregiver who may then abuse the senior. In the former it was noticed that some of the seniors who were abused were not dependent at all and that therefore there had to be more than vulnerability of the elderly victim to the equation. Researchers pursuing this line of inquiry embrace an 'exchange theory' in which the idea is that humans act to maximise rewards and minimise or avoid punishment. There is a co-dependency of sorts in which abuse arises because of anger of the carer who feels that they are not being rewarded for their efforts and that they depended on their elderly victims for such things as financial support and accommodation (which could be interpreted as significant 'rewards'. Local the reward often is the promise of inheritance which perhaps has not yet been ratified in a will.

The authors however note that all these theories are inter-related and give an 'integrated theory of abuse' in which caregiver stress, caregiver pathology, learned violence, environmental stressors, victim dependency/behaviour and victim pathology are all inter-related.

Political perspectives

The social context

Social work acknowledges that the elderly are a vulnerable group to reckon with; this is not obvious as it has only been recognised within the last thirty five years (Ife, 2012). Jin Ife argues that elder abuse can be physical, emotional or sexual but an additional category of abuse, the financial, requires specific human rights formulations, probably even specific legislation. It is a case of self-determination of one's property and financial affairs. He cites perpetrators can be unscrupulous sales representatives, financial advisors and brokers but especially from the person's immediate "family members seeking access to the person's savings, wealth or property either immediately through fraud and deceit or in the long term through pressuring the elderly person to change her/his will" (Ife, 2012). Ife also notes that there is an important difference between child abuse and elderly abuse: the mental capacity of the child improves as the child matures. The converse is the case for the elderly person where the mental capacity is more likely to decrease. Conversely helping elderly plan their future may 'pathologise' old age by focussing attention on the negative rather than the positive. He argues that this feeds into discrimination against the aging population. Policy can ignore the fact that many old people do not need help and are fully capable of conducting their own affairs. This only emphasises the need for social work to concentrate not only on the negative but also on what is positive about the aging process.

Nevertheless the vulnerability factor remains an issue and to use the same comparison that Ife uses with children, most children are raised in good environments and are not abused. The work done with child abuse by social workers has not undermined the positive developments in child development approaches and education of parents, schools and society. The emphasis should be therefore on empowering elderly people due to the fact, as argued in the introduction, that anthropologically we ought to recognise vulnerability as a human condition – something inevitable which society has an obligation to address.

Neutralizing vulnerability

Ten Have has argued that vulnerability poses a challenge of bioethics which has regarding vulnerability as simply a lack of autonomy, even though the Belmont report, which gave rise to the four principles of respect of autonomy, beneficence, nonmalefiscence and justice, address vulnerability in the first and last principles. Rather, as explained above, it ought to be seen as a human condition in and of itself.

Vulnerability is indeed one of the phenomena of human nature, and ought to be addressed by new principles. What values are being challenged? We see vulnerability not only in individuals but also in populations, and globalization has given rise to a greater understanding of its nature. Vulnerability is akin to human dignity and it is the main reason that politicians give, for example, to accept not only asylum seekers, but also those who tend to migrate for economic reasons. What is proposed here is an understanding of the implications of the ethics of fraternity and solidarity.

Vulnerable Persons Acts

Several countries have enacted Vulnerable Persons Acts which show the growing concern which the issue of vulnerability. Malta has started in this process by amending the law[2] on enduring power of attorney for those who have a power of attorney which formerly was useful only until the elderly person retains full capacity. Even though the underpinning philosophical discussion may not be addressed and Acts are devised to be seen through the lens of lack of autonomy of the vulnerable, it is a good start, although the social approach to vulnerability may indeed improve if we change our perception of its reality as has been argued here. What is needed however is a bio-psycho-social structure to look after elderlies' physical and mental well-being. Such an Act ought to include:

1. A procedure for reports of suspected and mistreatment
2. Education of the public and of the identified persons looking after the elderly individual
3. Safety plans which would ensure the safety at home of the elderly which go beyond telephone service[3]
4. Home visits by care workers and family doctors
5. In-depth assessment interviews on a regular basis

---

[2] *Civil Code (amendment) Act No. XIII of 2016,* (This amendment provides for the protection of vulnerable and elderly people from abuse from those who have power of attorney).

[3] Thus, for example, the carer can have cameras installed to monitor the elderly when they are not present. Moreover internet facilities can play a greater role. Already an EU COST Action (Shield-On, CA 16226) proposal is to study the living conditions of the elderly to make them more safe.

6. Ensuring contact with other family members and friends
7. A Support Network including the guardian, interested family. members, social workers, appointed family doctor, an appointed notary etc
8. A support network for the carer/s who are amenable to stress and who may not realise they are slipping into abuse.

At least elderly patients can be registered with their family doctor. When mentally sound, the elder person can be reassured that his or her general practitioner will always be called in and that, unless going through the support network, this doctor cannot be changed by the carer/s. This would avoid problems of competing interests when the carer calls his or her own general practitioner for the elderly person, who, due to the vulnerable position, would have to accept a new doctor not of one's own trust and with whom one has not yet built a confidential fiduciary relationship.

Major decisions, like changing of doctors, spending more than a fixed amount, etc. need to have the approval of the support network who need to be all physically present in ad-hoc or regular periods. There is considerable concern over power of attorneys who have been known to manipulate people to change wills and/or use their pensions inappropriately. The support network must be given regular accounts of how money is spent. Ideally evidence-based studies ought to be done to show which are the issues that concern the local population most and address them accordingly. The assembly of these multidisciplinary teams which include guardians and other family members must have duties clearly outlined. This guarantees the Council of Europe's statement to:

> "Enable elderly people to choose freely their way of life and to lead an independent life in their usual environment as long as they want and as long as possible, with:
>
> - housing that corresponds to their needs and their state of health or adequate help to fit out their house;
> - Medical care and services corresponding to their state" (Delperee, 2001)

This will see that vulnerability be treated as an ontological state of human beings, a state we will all pass through if we live long enough, and a state which is *natural* and which obliges us with an ethical duty as to the care of children whose natural state is accepted more readily. Elderly can be seen as a burden, especially now that this sector of the population is on the rise and governments encourage relatives to look after them. Even in health care we recognise the need for special training for those who work with elderly people. Financial benefits are not enough and support and training of the carer is important as well. Abuse has been seen to be also a result of stress and lack of recognition both by relatives, and the elderly themselves who, knowing they will leave some inheritance, believe they may have ownership of the carer. Abuse can be tackled easily in the beginning by recognising the pressure these people go through and providing courses, seminars and support. Whilst recognising that negligence and abuse can be premeditated, one has to recognise the difficulty of people looking after an elder member of the family when they have had no training, experience or knowing and find themselves suddenly in a situation which can also cause helplessness (and ontological vulnerability) on their part.

References

Bronowski, J. *The Ascent of Man*¸ BBC Books, UK, 2011. (Broadcast as a series on the BBC in 1973).

Delperee, N. (2001). European socaila policy for the elderly. In D. N. Weisstub, D. C. Thomasma, S. Gauthier & G. F. Tomossy (Eds.), *Aging: Culture, health and social change* (International Library of Ethics, Law, and the New Medicine, Vol.2. ed., pp. 125-119-139). Dordrecht, New York, Lonodn: Kluwer Academic Press.

Dyer, C., & Ostwald, S. (2011). Aging and health: Managing co-morbidities and functional disability in old people. In I. Stuart-Hamilton (Ed.), *An introduction to gerontology* (pp. 87-125). Cambridge, New York, Madrin, Melbourne, Cape Town: Cambridge University press.

EndCare (Erasmus+) Project, *Harmonisation on End-of-life Care*, University of Malta, 2016 (www.um.edu.mt/ms/endcare)

Englund, H. (2009). Human rights and moral panis: Listening to popular grievances. In M. Goodale (Ed.), *Human rights. an anthropological reader.* (pp. 209-228). United Kingdom: Wiley Blackwell Publishers.

Fluehr-Lobban, C. (2015). Anthropology and ethics. In D. Fassin (Ed.), *A companion to moral anthropology* (pp. 103-114). United Kingdom: Wiley Blackwell Publishers.

Gambino, G. (2017). Care and justice. In I. Carrasco de Paula., V. Paglia & R. Pegoraro (Eds.), *Virtues in the ethics of life. XXII general assembly of member of the pontificial academy for life* (pp. 103-114). Vatican City, Rome: Pontifical Academy for Life.

Gawande, A. (2015). *Being Mortal. Illness, medicine, and what matters in the end.* London: Profile Books in association with Wellcome Collection.

Gordon, R., & Brill, D. (2001). The abuse and neglect of the elderly. In D. N. Weisstub, D. C. Thomasma, S. Gauthier & G. F. Tomossy (Eds.), *Aging: Caring for our elders* (International Library of Ethics, Law, and the New Medicine Vol. 2. ed., pp. 203-218). Dordrecht, Boston, London: Kluwer Academic Press.

Ife, J. (2012). *Human rights and social work* (3rd ed.). Cambridge, New York, Melbourne, Madrid, Cape Town: Cambridge University Press.

Mallia, P. (2012). In Ten Have H. (Ed.), *The nature of the doctor-patient relationship. health care principles through the phenomenology of relationships with patients* (1st ed.). USA: Springer.

Mallia, P. (2014). In Ten Have H. (Ed.), *The nature of the doctor-patient relationship* (Springer Briefs ed.). Dortrecht, New York: Springer.
Nutik Zitter, J. (2017). *Extreme measure. finding a better path to the end-of-life.* New York: Avery.
O'Mahony, S. (2016). *The way we die now*. UK: Head of Zeus Ltd.
Ten Have, H. (2017). *Vulnerability. challenging bioethics.* London and New York: Routlegde.

Chapter 5
Community homes for the elderly

Among the many services offered locally for the elderly are services at home, and homes for the elderly. This chapter will focus on the latter and the experiences gained from it. It is in the last couple of decades that private homes for the elderly started to flourish and this is enhanced by the private-public partnership (PPP) initiative. Before that, going back three or four decades only St Vincent de Paul Residence (SVPR) seemed to be enough to cater for our elderly populations.

As the population grew various governments improved the wards, and built new building and enhanced the surroundings. The building of a Clock Tower had indeed caused some outcry for funds; but looking back why should we not have a nice place for our elderly. When we go back further, the place was referred to locally as 'Tax-Xjuħ', in perhaps a derogatory fashion. Even the place where it is was dubbed as a name, 'L-imgieret'. So, 'tmur l-Imgieret' could even be used jokingly, even if politically it ought to be incorrect when addressing an older person. Having said that some may still jokingly refer to themselves as 'tajjeb għall-Imgieret'. The place was also called Ħas-Serħ in the Labour Government of the 70's and 80's; as was fashion by this government to call other places with the prefix (or article) 'Ħas- or Ħal-, as in Ħal-Tarxien' as we use for villages. Thus Ħal-Tmiem, comes to minds. 'Ħal' derives from 'raħal', meaning village. In effect Ħal-Tmiem was a kind of village for tourists or people in transit. It did not last long. When it comes to the elderly Ħal- was a good term as it indicated a community rather than a village. Whether the concept of a community however can actually be achieved in such a place, or indeed, whether it is appropriate to call it such when it does not have the inherent structure of a commuiy – one of the most important is neighbours and people who have known each other for years', is doubtful and perhaps an over-reach in our fantasy.

SVPR at first was SVPH, the H for Hospital soon being replaced with an R for Residence, as was appropriate to call it. Nevertheless it continued to have full medical attention with on-call doctors and ward rounds. This is perhaps necessary for continuity and because there is no coherent and perfect plan yet found to work for us. The elderly live longer (although this does not mean they have a good quality of life), even if bed-ridden because they are drug-ridden with all the new pharmacology. Of course it would be ageism not to do so. But questions do come to mind if we prolong life without it being able to be fulfilled to a certain degree. Is this not what we mean by Active Aging, after all. A therapeutic approach would be more effective, if not efficient, as it includes other methods of rehabilitation and occupation than merely prescribing drugs. This chapter explores some of the issues. To be clear it is not a criticism; as at the end of the day we get what we pay for, but as an observation made by a mere doctor still serving his community as a general practitioner and indeed happy to be able to continue to see his patients within the same village or those attaching.

We need realistic goals for our elderly. Those of us of an age when we see our own now elderly parents entering a home quite quickly, in many circumstances put away the thought that they can put their minds at rest. They quickly find out that elderly, perhaps inherent to the health care professions, from carers, nurses to managers and visiting doctors, treat the elderly in a different way as we shall see. It is important however to notice that there are different categories of people who live in a 'Home', which seemingly is synonymous to a 'nursing home' in Malta, with few exceptions. In fact, the PPP Principle worked very well. On the one hand the government invests because it has the responsibility to look into the care of our elderly population; on the other hand business investors can be encouraged to build because the government will promise to pay for a certain amount of beds. What we need to be certain of are two factors. The first is that the elderly population will conitinue to increase; the second is that it is giving us a glimpse for those of us who are in their 50s to 60s as to what we can expect. Those younger may not be old enough to appreciate how close to them it actually is too, in the larger scheme of things. We need to think of this Future Generation of elderly, which are us. So it is meaningful to ask oneself – do I wish to be in a home; or what would I expect. This is not only non-selfish, but it also helps as a community to think about others as in thinking of how an ideal home ought to be, one is thinking about those who either do not have the time or for some reason do not think about it.

To start, there are various categories of residents. The first one should mention are those who choose to enter a home at an early age. They are usually in their 70s and go there to rest from daily chores and perhaps have an 'active-living' sort of life, being able to come and go as they please, have their food, cleaning, services ready and even though they forfeit a large part of their pension, they can count on no electricity expenses, which include air-conditioning throughout the year – warm or cool. Moreover, they do not need to bother about cleaning, cooking and can even have help with medication, washing and other activities they are incapable of doing. Some even continue to go to their home to water their plants and to feel independent. This may be the wisest option but certainly not the one more frequently taken. It is not the same in the United States, for example, where many elderly couples at that age go to warmer climates either in communities, with their own house with a pool (Florida is very popular), or go to other forms of residential areas with apartments or condominiums. It is doubtful if Malta can have such places unless one forfeits the principle of equity. But it is a possibility for those with enough savings and perhaps a property to sell.

The second category would be when a person needs to go into a home and the spouse decides to accompany the person. Although no statistics are available it seems that it is more common for a husband to accompany a wife rather than the opposite. Certainly, I have seen plenty of the first in my area and none of the second. Perhaps it is also because husbands die earlier. But there are cases which can break one's heart. I recently witnessed a patient with mild dementia and who quietly spent his days in bed but who could have been taken care of by community nurses; the wife refused to have nurses in her home and her daughters had to agree. Conversely, I admire an elderly woman who at first wanted to find a home for her husband who had advanced dementia (there were not community homes at the time in the area), as she was unable to cope. When visiting her home, one noticed that he was a very quiet man, older than his wife, but quite lean. When I explained the community services available and the burden of having to visit him at SVPR she readily accepted and he died peacefully at home several years later. She found fulfilment in this and it showed and expressed her gratitude.

However, there are those who are put into a home because of their dementia. The reasons vary from living alone without supervision to living with relatives who cannot cope. Although there are day-nurse services, one still has to pay a substantial amount for these and unless there are a number of siblings, it may not be affordable. To give an example, a family whose mother is 85 years old has moderate to severe dementia. She has four children. It costs around one thousand euros a month to have a 24 hour carer (and not all of them are willing to take them for walks, or do the washing), and one has to give them one-month a year paid leave and every two years, as usually they are foreigners, they have to pay for a one month holiday to their country. The government however pays for half, and four siblings can afford between one hundred to one-hundred-and-fifty euros per month each. Conversely if they are only two, or even worse, one, this probably makes it improbable and the only solution would be to go into a home; quite often against the elderly person's wishes but knowing that there is no alternative. This category also includes people who have relatives but who have ailments such as heart disease, severe arthritis, cancer, fractures etc., who cannot cope with daily living conditions, even though they can be visited by relatives every day.

Finally, there are those with severe dementia who need special wards and many of these community homes have special floors for these. It is indeed much better than the old dementia ward of SVPR. Having said that they have excellent one-to-one care there which modern homes are not able to afford. But the aesthetics is better (at least for those who visit them). There are no locked gates and the ward odour is usually better.

Whilst there are other reasons for entering a home, including younger people with severe disabilities, these constitute the major number and suffices our purpose here.

The home

The new PPPs are very modern, kept clean, have relatively good nursing care and carers for help with toilet, washing etc. They are run differently but generally they have a manager and one or two senior nursing staff. For the most they have fewer Maltese nurses and carers and most are foreigners (mostly from India and the Philippines). We shall not enter the political argument for this commodity, as it is a European-wide issue. Suffice it to say it has caused a further rightening of some centre right parties as it is seen not merely as serving people in need of asylum, but an economic need to keep salaries of the low-income level down. Moreover there are also less and less people willing to work in this sector, first because of the higher educational levels and secondly because salaries are what they are and also reflect a meaningful income according to your education. If you have a degree to become a health carer and this does not make significant change to those who do not have a qualification, then of course people will shy away from this work.

Some problems and some solutions

Physiotherapy

Homes are served by health centres. If someone has a fracture, then a physiotherapist will visit periodically but the actual physio-work is handed over to the carers. This reflects a need for a daily presence of physiotherapists. When one has a mother or father who has suffered a fracture and who require daily physio such as using a walking frame, and relatives see that this does not happen on a daily basis, let alone given further encouragement which results in wheelchair-ridden people who could have walked again, this give rise to some concern. The issue is that health care professionals such as nurses and, in this case, physiotherapists, are not numerous enough and perhaps it is time to think about equivalent salaries to that of doctors, who notwithstanding their more difficult and intense training, will have great opportunities and perks in the future. The solution of course is that we need to think about resident physiotherapist. One per home is certainly not enough and one needs to calculate the average number of fractures, strokes, and other needs and derive a suitable working-number of physiotherapist per amount of residents. Carers, can *then* continue to help under their supervision.

Files

Not all homes have physical files. Some have computer files but do not ask you to make an input when you see the patient. The physical folder still works best unless you want the general practitioners to keep walking for the bed-side to the counter to make notes. This wastes time and raises costs. It certainly takes more time to visit someone in a home than to visit someone in the patient's own home. Files of patients are not there only for the doctor to remember the history and details of the patient; what was the last treatment and dose given and when, for example. They are there for other reasons. The first being so that in the absence of the main doctor, any other doctor can know important things about the patient and what treatment etc., they have been given. Secondly if the patient is referred to hospital, the home can send the file with the patient for good continuity of care. Finally there is the medio-legal reason. Should someone complain, there is the written record on the file which explains reasons why or why not something was done.

To illustrate a clear example, this book has some chapters on end-of-life situations. Recently a 91 year old elderly woman developed a large lump in her groin in one of the homes. At that age it is unlikely that a surgeon would operate, especially because of her heart condition and dementia. I discussed with the family that one can send her to hospital for investigations. This would mean a change in her environment, blood tests done daily, and the works; only to be told at the end whether they will take the risk of operating on her as she may die during the operation. Moreover should they offer chemotherapy, were they willing she go through the trauma of nausea, discomfort etc? These are decisions which, if the patient cannot make, are to be decided by the family. I asked the daughter, (close to her 70s) to bring her siblings and together they decided that it would be better to keep her comfortable. One would be surprised at how more resilient elderly people are when they are left alone. Many interventions, exposure to hospital transport, procedures and indeed infection, etc can send them backwards. She may also pass away due to another condition rather than the tumour itself. They decided to keep her in the home. I left them a ticket of admission to hospital in case they changed their mind and wrote everything in the file, and as practice in this situation they signed the consent to the decision. When she was once taken to hospital due to an abscess (an infection of the lump with pus inside) the doctors agreed with their position and read the file. They cleaned the wound and gave antibiotics.

It is important to note that they did clean the wound and give antibiotics. The decision not to treat the cancer does not mean she should not get other treatment. I am often stopped by health professionals asking me why a 90-year-old on the do-not-resuscitate (DNR) order was given blood transfusion by the doctor. DNR means DNR, only. It does not mean do not give transfusion. These decisions are taken individually.

Communication

Communication between the resident/attached geriatrician and the general practitioner (whether attached or that of the patient) is not well organised in many homes. If someone decides to change a medication or to stop a treatment given by another one, the least the resident specialist geriatrician can do is call the family doctor and explain why. This frequent does happen but less often than ideal.

Conversely the communication with the nursing staff should be in writing. Staff change shifts and unless there is a going handing-over it is not done. This is a very frequent complaint of relatives visiting their parents. In one case a fracture of the hip was accompanied by a fracture of the wrist. Following a change in shift one carer pulled the patient from his arms, not knowing there was a fracture and the patient had to be sent back to hospital for the injury.

As everywhere lack of communication is what causes most problems. It is good policy that most homes do call the relatives when there is a problem immediately, informing them, for example that their mother fell but that there were no injuries and that she is well (or otherwise). This avoids confrontation and 'why-was-I-not-told' complaints. We now depend on many foreigners coming to Europe to work at various jobs. Due to lack of nurses, or lack of incentives to become a nurse, many foreigners come to European countries to work. Let me make it clear that we should be thankful that we find these people to help us; without them we would be in a much more difficult position. But like with every good thing come problems. Although they are given briefing and training, they come from different cultures and also different *clinical* mentalities. For example I had to explain to one of them why for a dying mother-of-three, who was 83 years old and had been admitted for sepsis (diffuse body infection) twice to hospital, we again discussed that this would go on interminably and finally she will pass away. What did they wish – to keep her comfortably at the home or to send her to hospital? They agree that it was the last hospital admission, especially the trip back to the home which sent her into a confusional state and then into an unconscious one. We decided to keep her in the home. We did administer a small dose of antibiotic and morphine but when asked by the nurse about a naso-gastric tube, I said no. She was taken aback. I explained later that dying people to not eat or drink if they are unconscious, and also if they are semiconscious sometimes. It is nature's way. There is no point in extending life by artificial means by a few days or even weeks to prolong the agony – after all feeding means that the food will need to be digested by a dying body and this may cause discomfort. The evacuation may not take place and cause further discomfort. Guidelines today oblige us to recognise that a person is dying, say, within the week. This is a clinical decision based on the situation of the patient, the result of blood tests on several organs, and indeed the state of the patient. Morally we can also administer morphine to relieve the pain and discomfort even if this shortens life, as explained elsewhere in this text.

Care for special cases

There are special cases of individuals. These include:

1. The blind
2. The deaf
3. The person always calling for a nurse
4. The sick
5. Common fractures, etc

When a person is sick, has come from hospital, has a fracture, the immediate attention is often formidable. As time goes on, as explained above the person with a fractured hip is helped and fussed about less frequently going down to almost zero.

There seems to be no protocol on how to deal with blind people; they need help with switching on the television. With today's technology many still need to ask their kids on how to change a channel from Netflix to television, let alone the blind who wish at least to listen to the quiz programme. Many do not know the basics that a blind person needs things – from chairs, to items on the table, to be left in the same place. They can trip on a chair that has been moved and they can search for a glass in vain only to hit it with the side of their hand and drop it on the floor.

The need for occupational therapists to help not only older people who have lost their vision but also to train nurses and carers on how to manage their environment is important. This requires attention to details. It is important perhaps to try to deal with this across the board, as not only blind people will prefer to have their stuff left where they put it.

One major problem some homes have is the handing-over process. Some do it excellently; some not at all, or shoddily. In one instance a man of 86 fell and broke his hip and the forearm of the same side. When returned to the home, everyone knew about the hip (somehow, because a hip fracture is common in the elderly, they were more aware of this than the arm). Following a change in shift one carer came to put him into bed and pulled him from the fractured arm, displacing the wound again.

Maltreatment and discipline

Unfortunately, due to the lack of finding staff; the lack of proper training and up-to EU level qualifications, different temperaments and cultures, there are situations of either maltreatment or indeed abuse of time. A study should be done, for example, to ask the relatives about the following:

- Have you ever found out that your relative was maltreated, shouted at, handled badly?
- Have you heard whether people offer money to staff (which of course discriminates against others or at the least confers preferences)?
- Have you noticed times when there are no staff on the ward, e.g. between lunch and tea-time, or, between 2300hrs and 0300hrs?

It is not that these things may not be expected to happen. But when they do the complaints should be handled well and not in a defensive manner. Since justice has to be done and seen to be done, it is important that relatives know as well. In one instance a patient dropped his bowl of soup which was left on his table. Before going to bed he accidentally knocked it on the floor and called the carer asking if they could clean it. The carer said that at that time they did not have a cleaner but said he would see what he could do. A person, (probably a cleaner), did come in and got angry at the patient saying that that was not soup but vomit! He shouted at the patient and covered the liquid with a towel and left. The mess was cleaned the next morning. The relative informed the management of this. They said that they would look into it. Later they told the relative that they handled the situation but said that they would not tell him what was done. As a relative of this person one would certainly wish to know whether he or she got suspended, sent away (as certainly no-one who shouts at patients and leaves the place unclean and in danger of slipping, should be working in a home. One need not know who the person was but it is quite legitimate to know that severe action was taken.

On a different and more general level, even those persons who can go to the toilet but need some assistance are often, given the workload, put on nappies and when they need to 'go' are told to 'go' in their nappies. '*Agħmel fin-nappy*' has become an all-too-common phase one hears. Does anyone wish to be treated like that. Given the workload this is understandable and some homes do indeed try to cater as much as possible to take the relative to the toilet when possible. It is only the carers who care about the dignity of the older person who see this as not only their duty but even perhaps going the extra mile.

Admittedly some elderly are very difficult to handle. After all they are elderly, come from a different period than young people, may be frustrated that they are in a home, dependent, and unable to 'live' as before. They probably know they will die there and they have no future to look forward to and are lucky if they get at least one visitor per day. But this may still frustrate the carers and nurses and sometimes they have to take action in order to control behaviour. It is this control that should be screened and noted in the file for medico-legal purposes:

- Who needs this treatment?
- For how long?
- What are we going to do?
- Handing over?
- Is there a system to document and report?
- Is there accountability?

For example one patient continuously shouting for a carer or nurse was given sedation. Everyone was happy. But the decision had to be communicated well between shifts and warned not to exceed the agreed upon management. Shouting at a patient is always degrading and not really good for the feel-good-factor in a home – after all it is a home, not a prison.

The government

The staff organisation and management

There are guidelines produced by the public sector in order for the private partnership to follow. These need to be updated regularly and clearly. One thing which one may point out here is that the management of homes varies from one to another. Private sectors may have their own way. Clearly however their are condition the government should impose. Some examples include:

1. One should have a nursing officer (manager) or a deputy at all times of each floor or ward or number of residents or dependencies.
2. There should be no time when you cannot find anyone – either carers or nurses; this occurs during times of breaks and during times of the change in shifts. Someone has to be available. This is often seen by relatives. "I could find no-one to speak to at the time I went".
3. Management should be divided into the clinical side and the hotel side. A general manager cannot do either and has to be on top to look, hear and indeed, as one patient pointed out sarcastically, 'smell' the situation. Conversely the clinical manager may be very good at her job but not so good when managing the 'hotel' part (as it is call) of the home – from

laundry, cleaning, maintenance, food, etc. The clinical manager cannot be burdened with these matters and must see that order is kept and that everyone knows to whom they are answerable. With different cultures working together this is all the more important for harmony in the ward. Where you come from should not affect the nature of your work.

4. What kind of daily activities are available; these range from good regular ones to the ridiculous where some are treated like children given a rod with a magnet to 'fish' for a paper fish drawing on the floor. It may be good for therapy but not as entertainment (at least not for all). What activities are there for those short of hearing, or for the blind? Contrary to what many think, the elderly are not there to 'rest', as the older saying goes – although some may be. If we are focussing on active aging we should be thinking not only about the monthly or weekly activity, which are usually done, but how people, even those with disabilities can keep themselves occupied during the day. One resident with experience in management was approved to give some advice; another was helped with an initiative to do a marathon. Yet another with experience in exercise offered to do exercise classes. This may not be within the regulation of the home unless done by a qualified professional, but they certainly can help in the organisation. Being told that they can watch the daily exercise programmes on their television is not really conducive to fostering an active and satisfying day.
5. Standard and regular training and updates for staff. Even terms meant in a good sense sound silly at times – such as '*sabiħ*', or '*sabiħa*'. They are nice, but only if offered to everyone – even to that person who makes a lot of noise or the problematic ones. It is not a reward. Also, it may not be proper sometimes and one may need to review the correctness in time. Moreover, are there updates on standards of care such as making an informed choice; when a relative requests a power of attorney document, do the homes 'stay out of it' or should there be some form of attention for abuse as is done in the public homes? What standard Continuing Professional Development is necessary.
6. Consistency of services. Let us use nappies as an example. One

> home may have a shop, and this may create a conflict of interest. If someone is getting free nappies from the government, why should they be made to buy from the shop if for some reason they are used up. Some homes take care of the procedure to procure the nappies themselves; others ask the relatives to do so. When nappies run out it is common to use those of others until the supply comes and is replaced; but if the home has them for sale and the relative somehow delays, would it be right (and ethical) simply to take nappies from the shop and charge the relatives. These conflicts of interest have to be addressed. Elderly have pensions and they need them for extra medications. Antibiotics, paracetamol, gels, etc are not given freely any longer. The 'pink card' has been almost phased out. Perhaps it should be introduced again for the elderly and pensioners.

In a PPP, the government is buying a service and has a right to insist on certain standards such as the above.

There are other issues which in time hopefully can be dealt with. We have improved from having 'wards' with six to eight beds with a maximum of two per room, sharing a bathroom. This has its problems of course. One need not go into details but characters may not agree; one may be dominant over the other; one want the TV on while the other does not; the toilet is not cleaned after one uses it when the other need to use it immediately afterwards, etc. We should be thinking about the future of having single rooms. Only a little more space is actually needed. Why does one have to be disturbed when there are the relatives of others. To be sure, there are people who are happy in a double room and the option can be kept. They may enjoy the company of others and their relatives. But the converse is frequently the case.

Chapter 6
The care of the elderly patient[1]

Old age requires special understanding of, feeling for, interest in, and commitment to the medical problems encountered. The family physician has children at one end of the spectrum of patients he sees and the elderly at the other. General practitioners often develop a fondness for their elderly patients. Old people are more committed to the family doctor of their choice and the fiduciary relationship they develop is especially strong. The general practitioner often becomes the 'life saver' for them and once one obtains the trust of an elderly patient, it is difficult to lose it. Elderly people seem to have an extra sense to know who really wishes them well and is interested in their welfare.

Western Europe, including Malta, has experienced a large increase in the proportion of the elderly population. This has been due to falling fertility rates and falling death rates due to improved living standards and health care. It is wrong to say that people are living longer. Of course there is more attention and understanding of the needs of elderly people. But medicine has progressed across the board, improving standards in all age groups. The falling death rates were seen especially in childhood and infancy. Many used to die in these aged groups particularly due to poor living conditions. Therefore, the proportion of people living has theoretically increased. This is coupled however with the fact that couples have less children. The overall effect is that we have a higher proportion of elderly, and consequently a lower proportion of people who pay national insurance in order to be able to provide adequate social services for these elderly, including pensions. Politicians have often discussed the implications this will soon have.

[1] Mallia, P. "Care of the Elderly Patient", in Mallia, P. *You and Your Doctor*, Chapter15, pp. 143-162. Agenda Publishers, 2006.

Suffice to say that in the past Dr Anthony Fiorini and I have argued for a separate operation list for elderly in order not to allow them to wait so long. Two years at the end-of-life is proportionately longer than two years when you are thirty. But in all fairness one has to keep the working population working in order to fulfil the needs of the same people of old age.

From the medical point of view, longevity sounds very much like a blessing. We all wish to live long so long as we are not a burden to others. And this is in fact whether old age is indeed a blessing or a curse. If we can add life to years, rather than years to life, and if therefore the quality of life is good, then old age is not a burden. But the body *is* aging, and we do not remain what we were before. So with this blessing comes a decrease in functioning and a myriad of different problems.

Some cell, most notably those of the central nervous system, the heart and the kidneys, do not divide. They must last a life-time. Therefore they age with the person and their efficiency decreases with the passing years. This is why there is so much ado about stem cell research. If we can give embryonic stem cells to people in some way, this may restore certain specific tissues, in the nervous system say, curing conditions like parkinson's and other neuronal disorders. But stem cell come at the expense of embryos, which therefore poses considerable moral problems.

There are many changes which occur in the body of an aging person. Much of the connective tissue becomes stiff and there is loss of elasticty. This causes wrinkling of the skin, stiffness of tendons and changes even in the lens of the eye. The bodies' immune system takes a plunge and moreover there is an increase in autoimmune disease; that is when the immune system turns again cell of the body itself. Overall there is therefore a decline in function, which although can be alleviated considerably by a healthy life-style, especially earlier on in life, which includes a good diet and regular exercise, will always to some extent be there.

Care for the elderly is different therefore than the normal check ups which adults ask for. Rather than a myriad of tests, the family doctor pays special attention to *functional assessment* – that is assessment how the person manages the details of the activities of daily life. One pays attention to:

- Perceptual function
- Cognitive function
- Emotional function
- Gait (how the person walks about)

There are special features in the illness affecting the elderly:[1]

- Multiple pathology and causes
- Atypical presentation of illness
- Slowness
- Failure of fluid balance
- Rehabilitation and functional assessment
- Ethical issues

For example, an elderly lady can have poor vision, poor gait due to osteoarthritis of the hip, suffer from a drop in blood pressure when she sits up from bed, have urgency to go to the toilet due to bladder instability, and above all else have an environmental hazard, such as a rug which may slip, close to the bed. This causes a fall when she gets out of bed in the haste to go to the toilet. Combined with her osteoporosis, the fall causes a fracture to her major legal bone. This in turn is another pathology which will then cause further problems. If the importance of preventing these circumstances (such as heeding the advice of the doctor to remove the rug; or to bring a comode close to the patient) is taken seriously and actively as the prescriptions one writes, families could prevent considerable distress to their elderly and themselves as carers.

Intellectual failure, incontinence, immobility and instability can all cause functional decline, even over a very short period. Moreover functional decline, such as inability to get out of bed, or taking to one's chair, or weight loss, may all be signs of serious illness, and thus present in an atypical way.

Left without care, an acute cardiac condition, such as pulmonary and lower limb oedema (fluid in the lungs and legs, which are caused by a weakening heart and which causes congestion), will lead to

[1] Coni, N., and Webster, S., *Geriatrics*, Blackwell Science, 2000: 25.

slowness nad weakness which in turn may render the patient immobile, dehydrated or confused, incontenent, or constipated. These can then cause a deep vein thrombosis or pressure sores, which could have been prevented had the original problems been attended to.

The greatest enemy I find is complacency because the doctor never really finds anything wrong. As soon as the frequency of the visits stop, the pulmonary oedema which was under control suddenly takes over. This may in turn cause a fall and a fracture. That the cause was the fluid in the lung may either be speculated upon in hospital or never really known, although the condition is surely to be treated.

The family doctor therefore looks for completely different things in the examination of an elderly patient[2].

GAIT

- Aided or unaided?
- Shuffling or striding?
- Stable or unstable?
- Difficulty in getting up from chair or sitting down?
- Parkinson's

FACE

- Parkinsonian
- Hypothyroid
- Anaemia
- Vitiligo
- Orofacial disorders
- Basal cell carcinoma
- Palsies

JOINT DISEASE

- Neck stiffness
- Shoulder pain
- Stiff hips
- Arthritis of knees
- Scoliosis (spine)

---

[2] *ibid.*, p. 27.

SELF-NEGLECT

- Dirty hands, face, body
- Dirty clothes, incontinence
- Unshaven face
- Unkempt hair
- Neglected nails

NUTRITION

- Obesity
- Under-nutrition
- Hydration

CONVERSATION

- Appropriate
- Short of breath
- Coherent
- Mood
- Speech
- Emotional lability

Special attention is then paid during the examination to heart sounds, pulses, bladder, and ankle jerks.

Contemplating surgery also is important in the elderly. One distinguishes between that which is obligatory, such as a carcinoma or a fracture of the leg, and that which is not. In elective surgery the main risk factors in the elderly are heart trouble, respiratory disorder, previous strokes, dementia, metabolic illness such as diabetes, overweight and frailty.

Disability and rehabilitation

Due to disease and injury, the elderly can suffer considerable impairment, disablility and handicap. An abnormality of structure from arthritis or function from a stroke, results in disablility or loss to perform activities in a normal manner. The ensuing disadvantages renders the individual handicapped to do normal daily activities such as cooking, housework, hobbies, and even dressing.

Rehabilitation is the restoration of the individual to his or her fullest physcial, mental and social capability. Despite continuing impairment, the individual can be helped to facilitate certain activities and much independence is obtained notwithstanding diseases such as parkinson's amputation, strokes, and fractures.

The family doctor plays a key role, if the family is wise enough to call him or her in early, to guide and motivate the patient. The rehabilitation services in hospital are adequate but maybe far from sufficient. Long waiting periods and waiting times in waiting rooms make many people, especially the most nervous and vulnerable, unwilling or unable to go and obtain the full benefit. The situation is much better at Zammit Clapp hospital, which offers a dedicated out-patient service for the elderly. However it is unfortunately unable to cope with all the population. Moreover, home visits are less available.

What can the general practitioner do. In the first instance the general practitioner can guide the family into using the government available resources optimally and motivate the patient, especially in time when one is losing hope. Many individuals who suffer a stroke for example lose the complete function of a limb simply because they do not understand the full benefits obtained from physiotherapy and the importance it has as the brain is trying to neglect that limb. Indeed, that is why maybe patients do not seem to care about the loss of function of the limb – the brain is in the process of excluding it. It is a survival mechanism. The person must be motivated continuously. Moreover, the doctor's advice, if heeded, can make an immense difference. Naturally the doctor will merely repeat what has been said in hospital, but repetition is key to motivating people and carers to do the useful, rather than what they feel is right. Many people, for example think they are helping their loved ones by helping them to dress, when in fact they are doing the worse thing possible as the disabled person will start to rely on them and not make concerted efforts in this critical period of time. Although one may think that as time goes by the person gets better, in fact they never will. I have a patient who has not completely recovered from a stroke which occurred three years ago because his wife insists on dressing and undressing him. Yet he is able to go up and down the stairs and go to his field where he spends a lot of time toiling and labouring alone.

This seems like a contradiction, but the help in certain activities has aided his brain in neglecting the 'lost' limb.

There are the obvious centres for rehabilitation. These include the hospital services, out-patient services, geriatric services etc. Then there are the not-so-obvious and private facilities. These need not be too expensive. When we consider the amount of money which is spend unwisely following such tragic incidents, the family doctor can help the family budget well their resources. For example, it may be wise to invest in some suitable furniture. Also sending for a private physiotherapist need not be that expensive, especially if a modest fee is charged. Therefore a two-month period of physiotherapy with three sessions a week at three euro per session, will cost between seventy and eighty euro (rates have increased considerably since time of writing). A price less than a hundred euro for a personalized services following such a tragic event is a bargain indeed when we consider we spend fifteen euro just to go to the hairdresser. Then it all depends on how important your health is to you.

It is important to realize that doctors have dealt with problems before. There is no such thing as 'nothing more can be done', or that one has to live with the condition. But it is also important to realise that depending on one's definition, almost 75% of disabled people in the community are elderly. Among these, the elderly-elderly (over 80), thirty percent become housebound often due to events which have quite abruptly withdrew them from the outside world, such as a fracture or stroke. The energy we invest in helping our elderly people in the community, especially if they are relatives, will add quality to their life and decrease the impact of people living in old-people's homes.

Dementia

The aging brain decreases by about twenty percent of its weight by age 90. The cells tend to shrink and there is neuronal (nerve cell) loss. Some have likened this to a withering fruit. A gradual decline in cognitive functioning is part of the normal aging process. However, marked confusion, disorientation, memory loss and other changes may signal developing dementia. Unfortunately, patients and caregivers may mistake the early symptoms of dementia for normal aging[3]. It is important to distinguish normal changes, which are benign and stable over time, from those that signal dementia which progress and render disabling over time. Approximately 75% of cases of dementia can be attributed to Alzheimer's disease[4]. Alzheimer's disease (AD) is associated with pathological changes in the brain. Other causes of dementia however can be vascular (blood supply to the brain) or may be attributed to other medical conditions, including depression (which is more common than usually thought of in elderly). Early intervention is thus important by the family members as soon as they detect any deterioration in cognitive function or behavioural problems. If treatment is started later, the deterioration is still slowed down, but the damage which has been done cannot be repaired.

For these reasons it is critical that people realise that the family physician can be made alert to the patient. The physician will elicit family concerns and promptly evaluate the situation. It is important to realise however as well that the medication which is available for dementia is very expensive and not available at the moment on the Schedule V free medicinals through the government. This reason is the high cost for these drugs. One of the best known is Aricept, which can cost just under a euro a day. Yet when one compares the suffering the individual and family endure once dementia starts to progress, and indeed the amount of money that is then spend, one can consider seriously budgeting for such important drugs. It is hoped that the best available drugs will become available through the health scheme.

It is important to understand the following points:

- Marked changes in memory are not part of the normal aging process and may signal dementia. Physicians may not always recognise the initial signs of dementia as patients may try to hide them. Effective diagnosis and management of dementia takes time; a typical 15 minute office visit is insufficient. Three separate visits may be necessary for accurate daignosis, with regular follow-up office visits (at least once every six months) to address and treat problems.

---

[3] *Diagnosis and Management of Dementia*, American Family Physician Monograph, 2001 (2); p. 3.

[4] *ibid.*, p. 4.

- By making a specific diagnosis as early as possible, the physician can suggest treatment plans and engage the patient and the family in decisions to plan the future. Recent evidence suggests that early intervention with available medications can slow the deterioration of cognitive function and the development of behaviour problems which helps maintain quality of life for the patient and caregivers and delays admission to a nursing home. Ongoing counselling with the patient's caregiver is essential. Although available medications can successfully slow cognitive decline and minimize disturbing behaviours, it is ultimately the caregiver" stamina that determines when nursing home placement will occur.[5]
- Mild cognitive impairment is now considered a strong indicator of AD and promptly diagnosing it correctly with initiation of therapy will slow down the progress. The physician will also have screening tests to detect dementia. The American Academy of Family Physicians suggest the evaluation of the patient with suspected dementia on three visits.

First visit

- A comprehensive history is taken, and a physical examination performed
- Immediate family members who have knowledge of patient are interviewed
- A Mini-Mental State Examination (standard test) is performed
- An assessment of family and caregiver needs is made.

Second visit

- Essential laboratory tests are made (these include a complete blood count, liver and kidney function tests, thyroid function tests, Vitamin B12 and folate levels, (HIV and VDRL tests to exclude HIV/AIDS and tertiary syphilis))
- Reassessment of family needs.

[5] *ibid.*, p. 3.

Third visit

- Review of laboratory tests and findings
- Discussion of treatment options, including costs, and follow-up plans
- Readdress family and caregiver needs.

There are both pharmacological and nonpharmacological interventions which can treat dementia and maintain a good quality of life, maximizing functioning and independence and to enhance cognition, mood and behavioural problems. The care is always patient-centred and the physician can educate the care-giver about the possible disturbing behaviors and how to be proactive. It would be good if there were support groups available as well. The family physician will ensure however that careful attention is given to the caregiver's health and mental status. This is something which probably only the family physician, and not the health center doctor, can be aware of, detect, and provide.

The evaluation and management of AD requires a multidisciplinary team, including the general practitioner, nurse and maybe also social worker. The family physician will coordinate this team. Other members of the team may be included as necessary, such as a psychiatrist, a psychologist, a nutritionist, a pharmacist, a podiatrist etc. Home consultations may be necessary which the general practitioner will organize. The most difficult for caregivers are the psychiatric and behavioural problems associated with dementia. These include personality changes, mood disturbance, agitation, delusions and hallucinations. Repeated questioning related to memory loss, restlessness, and maybe socially inappropriate behaviours as well. The family doctor is trained to describe the problems accurately, assess the patient, seek the possible causes and develop and implement a plan which can be reassessed and modified if necessary. Treatment may start with environmental changes and implementing behavioural changes, and may also involve, either immediately or at a later stage, the use of pharmacologic therapy. The latter is important especially if delusions, depression, psychosis and similar symptoms develop.

Finally, the family physician can coordinate advance directive that address situations in which certain treatment, such as cardiopulmonary resuscitation (CPR) can be withheld. This must be discussed with the patient and the family at the early stages, rather than during an emergency or when the illness has progressed to the point where the patient is incompetent to evidence a choice. Care for the elderly has become a speciality in itself and internal physicians have been specializing in this area. There are also diplomas directed to family physicians, especially those who have a lot of elderly people in the population they cover. But since family medicine has become a speciality, those who are legally able to say that they are specialists in family medicine will be in a good position to treat elderly and to distinguish the special problems which elderly people face. The field of geriatrics and gerontology shows conclusively how medicine has moved from treating immediate pathology to an awareness of the biological, psychological and social problems as well as to the medical. It is also a matter of prevention; recognizing instability in walking when one gets up from bed during the night may prevent a fracture which will render the individual bed-ridden for weeks and prevent considerable suffering. The family physician's job strategically leads him to people's homes and an assessment of the environment automatically forms part of the visit.

Chapter 7

Clinical intervention in aging: ethico-legal issues in assessing risk and benefit[1]

Risk-to-benefit analysis with or without concern for legal issues have always been the mainstay of clinical practice. 'Beneficence', insofar as a principle in medicine, has to a greater or lesser degree always been based on this issue. Even under the 'accusation' that what physicians called beneficence, was indeed 'paternalism' (and hopefully this argument is resolved and exhausted now), whatever decisions doctors used to take, was based on what in their opinion was in the patient's best interests and for the patients' good. Leaving patients ignorant of their disease and outside the realm of decision-making, was considered a therapeutic privilege and done in order to 'protect' the patient from news which he or she did not or should not know in order to keep them from grieve which could cause them more harm than good. Times changed and so did values. The word values is used in order to emphasis that it is not merely a question of relativism or simply because we understand human nature better. Rather it is because western culture cherished the concept of autonomy. It was indeed the philosophical debate which contributed considerably to increasing the 'principle' (in the Kantian sense) of respecting autonomy and trumping it over beneficence, until Beauchamp and Childress (1984) came around to give us, (or rather, lay down what was in the air), the 'four principles'. These evolved into an ethical framework and indeed doctors and health care providers were invoked to 'use' these principles in their decision-making, calling them *mid-level* principles. Principlism came under attack (as an example, see DuBose, Hamel, O'Connell, 1994) and the defenders went on to invoke methods of using principles,

[1] Mallia, P., "Clinical Intervention in Aging: Ethico-legal issues in assessing risk and benefit", *Journal of Clinical Intervention in Aging*, 2010:5; 373-380

such as specifying and balancing. There was not one principle to overrule the other. Specification and balancing were meant to address the particular situation, yet steering away from *situational ethics*.

Assessing risk and benefit would fall under the principle of beneficence. There is overlap also with the principle of justice as these decisions invariably also involve the use of resources that can be allocated elsewhere (without, of course, bowing to utilitarians, as indeed even a deontologist must make sure that he has a duty to society as well). In the meantime the field of gerontology and geriatric medicine has taken on new life. Rightly so, we are not only concerned with the elderly as a specific group, needing special needs with special attention to differences in medical care, just as children need a different approach to adult, but also because our populations, and perhaps cultures, are aging (Whitton, 2001).

Making decisions of risk-to-benefit for the elderly invariably therefore takes on a completely different dimension than adult, not only because where the elderly are concerned there is a different physiology and an aging body, but also because we are dealing with perhaps an aging culture, and more persistently so because we have to face the bottom line question: Is it worth treating this patient at this stage of life? Is it in their best interest? Is it in *societies'* 'best interest'? These may be blunt questions but it is a reality from which the discussions of end-of-life decision-making and cardiopulmonary resuscitation, and Advance Directives have arisen; from which we answer whether questions into research into longevity, to mention but one example. Since we are discussing an ethical concept, and not merely a clinical algorithm, what we have at base is our attitude, in philosophical terms, towards our elderly populations. We must distinguish what is common to all and how to deal with culture. This paper is divided into three parts, with perhaps some overlap. The first discusses the reality of principles as an ethical framework and whether in essence it is our values towards the above questions which define outcomes. Secondly, discusses three real-world situations. The third discusses how we view elderly in this post-modern society, for it is only this which can truly address clinical situations.

Why principles and why conflict?

I make no reservations for not being a principlist. Indeed, I admire the whole rhetoric it contains; neither am I a virtue-ethicist, who try to find meaning in virtues within these principles, perhaps bowing into religiosity and community at heart. I believe that all our decisions are based on our virtues. Alas, sometimes virtues change; sometimes we make compromises. But inherently we are what we are because we have basic learned concepts throughout life that then indeed give us our principles. But both the use of and the foundation of these principles are inherently attached to our virtues of what is or should be right and wrong. A difference at this level, and you invoke a different reasoning on how the same principles are used to arrive to another different answer. Indeed when we deliberate a moral problem we start with an empathic feeling of what is right and what is wrong. We then discuss the principles in defence of this. Rational thought of the situation may allow us to change our course and perhaps the final decision, but our initial value-system remains unchanged. Indeed we have conflict amongst principles because we have different value systems. Gregory Tillett (1999) perhaps best explains this.

Tillett, in his analyses of resolving conflict distinguishes three concepts, or categories, of differences between ideas, humans, relationships, or internal (within oneself) issues: Problems, Disputes, and Conflicts. A *problem* can be resolved by management – “by the agreement on how something can or should be done”. We can easily conceive of a difficult clinical situation in which one consultant or family practitioner asks the advice of another; doctors within a team discuss between themselves and with patients on courses of action, especially within a context where there is refusal of a particular kind of treatment. Tillett points out that problems can indeed become disputes and can disclose conflict.

A *dispute* occurs “when two (or more) people (or groups) perceive that their interests, needs, or goals are incompatible and they seek to maximize fulfilment of their own interests or needs, or achievement of their own goals (often at the expense of others)”. I recently experienced a situation which explicates this very clearly in relation to a decision for an elderly woman who was being taken care of at her daughter’s home. This daughter had three brothers, one of whom had distanced himself from his sister due to a dispute with her husband. The main issue was that this brother convinced the others that their mother should be put in a home because he refused to visit her at their sister's home. Of course, prima facie, the best interests of the patient was for her to remain at home. However, it transpired that the woman was very depressed because this son, who was evidently her favourite, was not visiting her. The undue pressure was indeed coercive, and the woman gave in to go to the home in order to be able to see all – not at all a voluntary choice. In the meantime she needed hospitalization. After eight months in hospital and no remedy in finding a place at an institution, the decision had to be reversed to take her best interests: fear of a hospital infection, which had become a great risk, had to be taken into account. Since the daughter was still willing to take her back, this course of action was taken, and the necessary legal procurements arranged. At each stage however a *value*-laden decision was taken, which brings us to the third category: conflict.

Conflict, again as defined by Tillett, "arises when two (or more) people (or groups) perceive that their values or needs are incompatible – whether or not they propose, at present or in the future, to take any action on the basis of those values". Whilst problems and disputes arise within specific situations, conflicts do not need one. Two parties can be in conflict because of beliefs or because of the values they uphold. Hence the heated debates on abortion, euthanasia, etc. But as in the case above, we may find that superficially, at least, the people involved have the same values – they all loved their mother – but when it comes to taking a decision which was in the best interest of their mother, it was rather a decision in their own best interests which had become evident, until a situation arose which gave enough strength to override these different values. The difference in value was between one in which X would rather have his mother in a home and be able to see her (and, perhaps that she would be able to enjoy him), and the same person admitting that notwithstanding that his mother would not be able to see him, his sister was in a better position to take care of her and that given the state of existing homes, she may be better off. Thus, a question of values and needs come in. The conflict was that between X and the husband and not the situation.

There admittedly can be a hazy line between a dispute, as this case had, and a conflict. One has to delve into the narrative of each participant in order to reveal a conflict and understand that the matter is not simply one of disputes. One can resolve the dispute and still not have handled the conflict, thus remaining 'hung-in-the-air', so to speak, as indeed was illustrated in this case, when the brothers agreed that the mother be allowed to go to their sisters' but on the condition that she use her pension only and not her savings in order to take care of her; if she needed a new bed or a commode, they were not willing to contribute either. This coercion reveals the underlying conflict between the daughter's husband and the dominant brother. Whether a question of needs or values, these were put above the needs of the mother or the value to respect and meets *her* needs. Certainly, this was not a dispute any more but a conflict, which unfortunately the medical practitioner or team may not be able to handle, unless by bringing in the law or referring them to some other form of therapy if they accpet.

Following Heraclitus, *Justice is Conflict* (MacIntyre, 1996). Doctors make decisions in the light of beneficence and at the same time doing justice to the person(s) and the situation at hand. By 'doing justice', we obviously do not merely mean that the situation is handled well and correctly (within, that is, the boundaries of standards of care), but we seek that justice is done morally. Deciding *whose* justice, and which rationality is certainly not easy in the modern sense, especially in dealing with end-of-life situations, whether to treat or not to treat, whether to leave elderly for acute treatment at their home, or incur a more expensive, perhaps better treatment, but in a hospital setting. Certainly there can be hardly a better exposition of this philosophical reality than that of MacIntyre's. Whether he does justice to the topic is probable; whether he resolves the dilemma is uncertain. Certainly he speaks extensively of *traditions*, which is "an argument extended through time" – it can be a medical tradition or a religious tradition or simply a tradition of horse-riding. However, what is certain is that sometimes, traditions come into conflict. And they come into conflict because of their values and how they view justice. I follow Solomon (1992) in agreeing that morality cannot be reduced to any strict Kantian system of principles. The very fact that the four principles of health care require further specification and balancing shows that a deeper sense of the real situation is needed – and what this usually boils down to is the *narrative* of the parties involved who bring forth their values and needs. Principles can help us define and understand more clearly the issues at hand. Solomon does not particularly like MacIntyre's use of traditions, in the sense that it still leaves open the nostalgia for religion and a sense of community, but goes on to admit, that Aristotle, did invoke a sense of community when speaking about virtues. Neither does he associate virtue with feminist ethics, values not being supposed to be held captive to gender, even though the feminist ethics may have a point in contrasting male principles which are hard, oppressive, and impersonal, with female virtues of warmth and caring. Values are universal. On the other hand that principles are irrelevant – in the sense of a person 'having no principles'. But colloquially by having principles we are actually talking about the *values* a person holds as well. Principles do indeed guide, but in themselves are guided by underlying values. If I have a so-called value for life and am not in favour of euthanasia, I invoke principles to leads me to this conclusion. Conversely if my value system of life includes terminating suffering even by allowing physician-assisted suicide, then I will use the same four principles to reach the opposite goal.

Clinical decision-making

Having summarised the philosophical foundations on which risk-benefit analysis is based here, relevant various clinical situations we are faced with in health care are grouped. Jonsen, Seigler and Winslade (1986) classify three forms of disease and goals of medicine that are summarized here with particular reference to care and decisions for the elderly. These authors say that, "physicians encounter disease in three forms. In the first, the patient suffers from an acute illness that, once diagnosed, can be readily treated and cured. In the second, the patient experiences a process that causes serious disabilities and which, while some relief can be provided, will progress despite treatment and eventually case death. In the third, the patient suffers a chronic disease that can be effectively treated so as to relieve many of the most debilitating effects." For simplicity they use the acronyms ACURE, CARE, and COPE. ACURE is an acronym for Acute, Critical, Unexpected, Responsive, and Easily diagnosed and treated; CARE stands for Critical, Active, Recalcitrant and Eventual and COPE for Chronic, Outpatient, Palliative and Efficacious. Perhaps using simply *Acute, Critical* and *Chronic* would have been quite an accurate substitute, but these acronyms serve the purpose just as well and are applied here.

Jonsen et al. point out that physicians habitually approach medical problems by attempting to determine the indications for or against medical intervention. They suggest that we face ethical dilemmas in the same way as well. In fact assessing risk and benefit takes both medical intervention and ethical dilemmas to task especially when considering elderly patients and when one asks oneself whether one should treat or not in a particular case. Medicine remaining a science of uncertainty, even these acronyms are taken by the authors to be understood as probability statements rather than absolute designations. Indeed uncertainty therefore makes good decision-making in the face of risk-benefit analysis, not simply one of clinical competence but also one which is value-laden, and therefore based on values and virtues.

Most goals of the medical encounter are of the first group. They are acute and relatively straightforward conditions, especially once a diagnosis has been made. The situations may be critical and unexpected, such as meningitis, reversible and easily treated (by easy one of course does not mean 'easy' in the strict sense, but that one knows what to do and has an immediate plan of action based on evidence-based medicine and/or standards of care). Ethical situations in this form of situation may range from simply refusal of treatment to families not wishing the elderly patient to know. Recent literature suggests a more cultural-sensitive approach in these clinical situations (Searight & Gafford, 2005; Crane, Wittink, & Doukas, 2005; Brody & Hunt, 2005), respecting the wishes which may be culturally sensitive. In Japan, for example, it may be considered lack of respect to let an elderly person know of the medical condition, with the sons and daughter taking on responsibility (*ibid.*)

The second category (CARE) describes patients with active, progressive and deleterious effects. One can easily see many elderly people in such situations, though by no means is it restricted to this section of the population only. Under this category lie most of the ethical dilemmas facing end-of-life decisions, such as withdrawing of life support, decisions not to intubate, decisions not to resuscitate, and irreversible coma/brain death. Issues of Advance Directive are also at issue in this category. So are the mainline ethical discourses of ordinary vs. extraordinary treatment, killing vs. allowing to die, treating vs. TLC (Tenderness, Love and Care) etc. These are situations that inherently carry the legal issues. How would we distinguish between passive euthanasia and allowing someone to die? What is in fact ordinary and extraordinary treatment? The standard of care comes in heavily. Even in invoking the principle of double effect by using high doses of morphine, for example, to treat palliatively, knowing that there is a risk that one may die of the morphine and that this was a foreseen but unintended consequence, one must understand the nature of increasing doses of morphine and not be caught in a dispute of hastening death by going about the principle of double effect. Indeed, even though the principle has four basic rules to it, it is heavily burdened on the moral agent to ascertain that it is morally and correctly invoked (just as it takes a moral agent, for example, not to abuse the Abortion Act in the UK). There is always a *standard (of Care)* in increasing dose strengths, although this is a patient-sensitive decision and hence can be externally seen as subjective.

There is no duty to treat when treatment is judged useless. There is neither a duty to treat when it is deemed extraordinary. Although today, 'proportionate' and 'disproportionate' are terms which may be used instead of ordinary vs. extraordinary, the latter are not only still the most commonly used terms, but they are probably the best guideline to make a judgement on risk to benefit. One must clearly understand the meaning of *extraordinary* however to make best use of the term and for this one must look at its original Catholic origins. Extraordinary means of preserving life are "all medicine, treatments, and operations, which cannot be obtained or used without excessive expense, pain or other inconvenience for the patient or for others, or which, if used, would not offer reasonable hope of benefit to the patient" (Kelley, 1958).

A closer look at this definition shows how this covers most, if not all, legal issues that may arise when making moral choices on risk to benefit. When assessing risk, we are indeed facing the particular and singular clinical picture of *this* patient. Fitness for operation, side effects and interaction of drugs, wishes of the patient, physical state of the patient, etc. The definition clearly does not take into account the state-of-the-art of medicines and technology and something that is considered extraordinary today, may by no means remain so tomorrow. Conversely something that is quite ordinary treatment in one country, either because of culture or economic status, may indeed be extraordinary in another. *Family* need not be put to excessive burden, especially if they are required to pay or to go through extraordinary measures to meet the patient's needs. Clearly, where insurance and state cannot or will not pay, the family cannot morally be held responsible to take all measures necessary (in Malta, it has almost become a societal pressure to go to the UK for care when one finds no hope on the island, even if consultants say that no further treatment can be found there). Of particular note is that even *medicines* and excessive expense are mentioned in the definition, and, pain or inconvenience to the patient or family. Hence a treatment which cannot be afforded or which will cause prolonged agony, need not be given. We are not merely speaking of *futile* treatment then.

The third and final category is that of COPE. These are mostly found in outpatient and in community settings of family practice. They deal with the chronic and the palliative. Although Jonsen et al. lament that the ethical issues here may be less evident, they in fact may pose the same issues discussed above. COPE is a good acronym because in fact we are working with the patient to 'cope' with the illness. Although the same goals of preserving life, preserving function and reducing pain and suffering are used, they take on a more patient-centred approach and reach compromises with the patient which allow him or her to participate in the treatment. Whilst there may be no drama as in life-and-death situations, there is a quality-of-life perspective and also end-of-life decision-making to face. The American College of Family Physicians have recently given much attention to helping families cope with end-of-life and also address the cultural aspects of individuals and families (Lang et al., 2005). This departs considerably from the earlier days of bioethics up till some time age where autonomy meant revealing everything to the patient and almost burdening the patient with information, giving details in order to allow them to feel they were making a choice, or preferably made the choice themselves. This cultural-sensitivity brings back the onus on the practitioner to be truly patient-centred and to share the burden, at the same time, with the patient – who usually indeed seeks the doctors' advice. The bigger burden lies with difficult patients: those who are non-compliant and those who pose problems such as never being fully satisfied. In these situations the doctor may be impelled to transfer the care to someone else, as a breakdown of the relationship is perceived to have occurred. Yet COPE nurtures strongly on the doctor-patient relationship and on compromise; this may in turn translate into breakdown occurring less. Legal issues may arise with the family who may not be satisfied, especially after the death of, the care of their parents. Documentation is medico-legally paramount. It is important to acknowledge in this regard however that the involvement of the family as a community-based approach to treating the elderly is still compatible with the patient-centred approach (Wicclair, 1999).

The social understanding of aging

Of course, the concept of aging changes. Do we meat the requirements, ethically, of an elderly man with erectile dysfunction, or do we retort with a statement about his age. Yet, many bioethics committees recommend against women having fertility treatment beyond their menopausal age. With advancing technology, the right to treatments, perhaps a future elevation of average mortalities, and hence further aging populations, we may have to give ground to the yearning of the elderly spirit to continue enjoying life beyond the social boundaries thus far accepted. Leon Kass, former chairman of the United States' Council on Bioethics, and a staunch Catholic ethicist, much as he is respected for his intellect and capacity to make people reflect more deeply about the crossroad of technology and ethics, found considerable opposition to his general wariness of reproductive technology and efforts to forestall aging (Weiss, 2005). His turbulent debates on the council were a probable cause in his stepping down as chair of the council and being replaced by Edmund Pellegrino.

A risk to benefit analysis cannot therefore not look at the social concept of aging in a post-modern, and perhaps post-human society. These changes may be sudden or slow but they will occur. The concern it is to us now is in making the same analysis of legality, risk and benefit not only to medical care but also to research, this being imperative to the advancement of medicine. We have to decide which research is moral and which not to finance with public funds. There are strong arguments for the moral imperative to further research on elderly subjects even though research in this realm is both "ethical required and ethically suspect" (Schafer, 2001). Do we carry out research in order to increase longevity, or to curb the aging process of the body, or even perhaps to stop aging all together? Whereas better cures and medical advances have already brought this out, it was never really a medical imperative. It was, at most, a welcome, though perhaps foreseen, consequence of treatment and care. Yet the line is quickly coming close which draws a distinction between a rise in the elderly population due to better survival and a deliberate search for survivorship and longevity through such research into the genome and molecular cell biology.

In discussing aging and the sociology of embodiment, Featherstone and Hepworth (2000) give an interesting account worth reflecting upon. At the end of the day, the body is the bottom line, when we survive to deep old age (Woodward, 1991). Elias, in his old age acknowledge with an air of almost awe that there is a 'simple reality' of a finite life (Elias, 1985). The 'body in decline' therefore, for Featherstone and Hepworth, is a central issue for contemporary society to come to terms with. They assert that this does not mean that historically, when life expectancy was much shorter, people did not strive to prolong their life. The fear of death, the intensity of bereavement, and the longing for earthly pleasures where all issues to take to task.

'It is precisely in the struggle to reconstruct this cultural inheritance of pessimism that the element of difference between past and present attitudes towards aging through the later period of the life course may be found (Hepworth & Featherstone, 1982; Featherstone & Hepworth, 1989). This reconstruction, according to these social authors, lies in moving away from the pessimistic and melancholic processes of aging to one of optimism and a period enriched with distinctive creative possibilities (Featherstone & Hepworth, 2000). Only in this way can the structure of feeling and attitudes towards aging be changed, especially with regards to the aging body. This 'social reconstruction' (although many disagree with social constructionism, and perhaps a better phrase would be simply to say 'a change in social acceptance'), will then perhaps illuminate our attitude towards caring for our elderly in a new way and not simply as seeing them as one of the group of 'vulnerable' populations, which indeed they may be. We may see new light in research into the elderly and perhaps even in some form of longevity and prevention of body decline, which would bring with it a change, or rather a continuation, of activity formerly done: from sexual, to educational and occupational. We are already seeing countries prolong the retirement age due to improved standards of living and quality of life; and this not merely because elderly populations are on the rise and we need to 'keep' them with our taxes.

In understanding our ethical and legal attitudes to the risk and benefits of treatment, we must indeed be wary therefore of any desire by groups, such as practitioners of geriatric medicine, to make claims over a specialized form of knowledge and to legitimate the imposition of controls over aging members of the population (Katz, 1996). One should not take this to mean that geriatric medicine should not exist; indeed it should exist to protect this sector of the population from this pessimistic attitude and turn it into the optimism being argued for. This entails a change in concept even of the discipline itself. It need be an 'advocate', much as family doctors are advocates for patients and do not see the family solely in their medical dimension but more consistently in the biopsychosocial dimension, acting as family counsellors and advocates for patient rights. Notwithstanding the discipline of geriatrics and notwithstanding the vulnerability an increased percentage this sector of the population experience, we cannot continue to see old age as a form of pathology and the body in decline as a medicalized reality, which according to Katz, medicine is accused of. Perhaps we need to understand that the 'stages' model of life is a cultural cliché' as are expression of 'ticking of the clock' (Gubrium, 1995).

Should we strive for technological advancement of aging?

"The implications for the sociology of ageing are clear: it is no longer possible to make adequate generalizations about the aging process that are grounded on biological assumptions about the ages of life. Nor is it particularly useful to adopt schemata of the life course based upon loosely conceptualised models of unspecified processes of interaction *between* the ontologically distinctive entities, body, self and society. As a consequence contemporary models of ageing into old age must be increasingly post-modern, by which we mean they must anticipate even more advanced forms of bio-cultural destabilization" (Featherstone & Hepworth, 2000). These authors eloquently argue how our struggle is not really with biological decline, but with the social constriction of aging that has been the centre of debate. Hormone Replacement Therapy (HRT) even if it had an element of success was more about 'remaining young and active', hidden behind the excuse of better heart and skin outcomes, until the reality of the cancer issue came to light – something which many were very sceptical about from the very beginning. The 'social pressure' of HRT cannot be denied – many women who sought a better skin complexion and less wrinkling sought it out solely for this reason. It is interesting that post-modern feminist studies into the interpretation of age, was associated with wisdom. Before Patriarchal societies, the female crone was seen as a naturalistic and matriarchal part of life; the wrinkles being badges of honour (Gree, 1991). History has brought about a separation of the self from the body and society; the seeking of youth is found at the base of this force. Whether it be the result of patriarchal influence feminism blames, is beyond the scope here. The profound reality is that it is an existential issue: and entity to be reckoned with. This dualism: the separation of the self from the body lies in the very nature of the fear of aging – a declining body. "If I were twenty years younger…" is an expression that perhaps was less heard in primitive society, which adorned their elders with a wisdom and respect much less seen today. This lies at the heart and concept of the recent change towards end-of-life decision-making. Western culture is learning yet again from populations which lagged behind the materialistic taint and preserve many of their traditional values: such is the case for eastern countries.

There is however a downside to this reasoning as well. It lies in the non-acceptance of current culture. Featherstone and Hepworth continue to make the argument that whilst accepting the limits of the body and the aging process as having its own gains, it adopts a negative attitude to technological advance in which medical intervention, such as HRT and other future possibilities are viewed negatively. Indeed the word 'fundamentalism' is often used in an accusatory fashion, in ethical circles, as opposed to 'relativism'. This war of words reflect do not reflect a dispute but a *conflict*. Thus the main question would be of the form: is HRT unnatural and a threat to womanhood? Indeed there is much sense in *not* seeing technology as an external factor to human nature, but as a relationship between nature and the human bodily nature (which created the technology itself), as a culturally dynamic process. We have stopped seeing technology as part of our nature – it is the human nature, which creates it just as a monkey uses a stick. Humans started to culture fire and materials from the beginning of their existential nature. Indeed they have the capacity of self-destruction. But we must have faith in the forces of our very nature to overcome this fear as well.

Treatment and 'medicalization'

When seen in this light, we must be forced to accept a change in balancing risk as opposed to benefit. Whilst medicine has been attacked of paternalizing and indeed dominating in a Foucauldian sense, the sociology of medicine, the truth lies perhaps somewhere else. It is the world in general which has strived for technology and improvement of the human condition. Medicine has certainly taken advantage of new technologies for better cure; but research is often not carried out by 'medicine' as such, but by corporations who strive to satisfy the thirst of society – and profit of course in the process. There is a delicate, and sometimes controversial, balance with cultural and religious values. Certainly we question to what extent do we want technology to influence the human condition. There is a nostalgia, a longing to remain attached to certain roots. But it is not acknowledged that these roots do not exist. Technology has been advancing for centuries; it is only that we are witnesses to a boom lately that surprises us. Hence the reality and emergence of the new field of bioethics, as opposed to the centuries' old Hippocratic tradition, written in a time when technology was also blooming but not to the extent of this post-modern society.

We may still be tied therefore to concepts of not treating the elderly because of their age. Do you treat a woman of 94 who has developed breast cancer? The balance between cultural non-telling, and indeed giving a treatment adequate to what the body can withstand (it would be unwise to opt for surgery, but certainly a long-term course of Tamoxifen, even if palliation is not needed) is not that difficult to conceive. Legally therefore we should attempt treatment, and withholding treatment because of age can be conceived criminal. Accepting however cultural criteria such as the children of this woman, indeed in their late sixties themselves, of not giving her the bad news, even if she had never explicitly said that in case of illness, she would not want to know, is the morally (and perhaps legally) right thing to do.

What is probably wrong in our approach to elderly is to see the changing body as a pathological process. Even if we can come to accept change in body parts, better appearance etc as socially acceptable, there will always be a time of reckoning with death and the human condition. Decline begins very early on in life – perhaps immediately after the peak when one is still beginning adulthood. There are certainly problems which affect the elderly more, as there are problems which affect children more. What we should not tolerate is the marginalization of the elderly; even though perhaps having separate wards or hospitals, as having hospitals for children, is a must. Socially many people in society are want to abandon their elderly or not see their well-being as a 'worth-while' process. Mallia and Fiorini (1998) have argued for separate surgical lists for elderly to enhance 'life to years' rather than 'years to life'. Two years for a seventy-year-old have a larger proportion of one's remaining life-span than the same number for a forty-year-old. There is a perception that the elderly may wait longer in certain systems for elective operations. One of the referees (anonymous) indeed pointed out that it would be a far better use of resources to operate on a forty year old family man, arguing from a productivity point of view. This kind of attitude has been carefully avoided in bioethics, even in utilitarian circles. It is here that legislation can help.

Conclusion

Certainly, balancing risk and benefit, may not work out in favour of the elderly person. A new social awareness towards aging helps cultivate an attitude that old age is worth for what it *is* rather than for what elderly *do* or what they *have*. Whilst looking at the risk and benefit of treatment, we cannot ignore the larger risk/benefit picture of what research and medicine hold in the future. Advanced research must be respected as part of human nature to ask, invent and discover. A balance must be struck to not uproot people from their cultures and this is what gives people identities. Simone Weil (1949) warns against uprooting people; cautioning that 'uprootedness' leads to misery and spiritual lethargy on one hand and to violent efforts to adapt and uproot those not already uprooted.

References

Beauchamp, T.L., Childress, J.F., *Principles of Biomedical Ethics*, 3rd Edition, Oxford University Press, New York & Oxford, 1989.

Brody, H., Hunt, L.M. "Moving Beyond Cultural Stereotypes in End-of-Life Decision-Making", in *American Family Physician*, February 1, Vol. 71(3), 2005: 429-430.

Coni, N., Webster, S., *Geriatrics*, 5th edition, Blackwell Science, Oxford, London, Edinburgh & Paris, 2000.

Crane, M.K., Wittink, M., Doukas, J.D., "Respecting End-of-Life Treatment Preferences", in *American Family Physician*, Vol. 72(7), October 1, 2005: 1263-1268.

DuBose, E.R., Hamel, R., O'Connell, L.J., *A Matter of Principles? Ferment in U.S. Bioethics*, Trinity Press International, Pennsylvania, 1994.

Elias, N., T*he Loneliness of Dying*, Blackwell, Oxford: 1985.

Featherstone, M. Hepworth, M., "Ageing and inequality: consumer culture and the new middle age", in D. Robbins, L. Caldwell, G. Day, K. Jones, and H. Rose (eds.), *rethinking Inequality*, Gower, Aldershot, 1996.

Featherstone, M. Hepworth, M., "Ageing and old age. Reflections on the postmodern lifecourse", in B. Bytheway, T. Keil, P. Allatt and A. Bryman (eds), *Becoming and Being Old: sociological Approaches to Later Life*, Sage, London, 1989.

Featherstone, M., Hepworth, M., "Ageing, the lifecourse and the sociology of embodiment", in Graham Scambler and Paul Higgs (eds.), *Modernity, Medicine and Health. Medical Scoiology Towards 2000*, Routledge, London & New York, 1998: 147-175.

Gubrium, J.F., *Individual Agency, the Ordinary and Psotmodern Life*, Open University, Centre For Aging and Biographical Studies, Milton Keynes: 1995.

Jonsen. R., Siegler, M., Winslade, W.J., *Clinical Ethics*, 2nd edition, Macmillan, New York, Toronto & London, 1986: 16-43.

Katz, S., *discipling Old Age: The Formation of Gerontological Knowledge*, Iniversity Press of Virginia, Charlottesville and London: 1996.

Kelly, G., *Medico Moral Problem*, St Louis: Catholic Hospital Association, 1958: 135.

MacIntyre, A., *Whose Justice? Which Rationality?*, Duckworth, UK, 1988.

Schafer, A., "Research on Elderly Subject: striking the right balance", in David N. Weisstub, David, C. Thomasma, Serge Gauthier and George F. Tomossy (Eds.), *Aging: Decision at the End-of-life*, International Library of Ethics, Law, and the New Medicine, Kluwer Academic Publishers, Dordrecht, Boston & London, 2001: 171-206.

Searight, R., Gafford, J., "Cultural Diversity at the End-of-Life: Issues and Guidelines for Family Physicians", in *American Family Physician*, Vol. 71(3), February 1, 2005: 515-522.

Solomon, R.C., *Ethics and Excellence*¸ Oxford University Press, New York & Oxford, 1993: 112-117.

Tillett, G., *Resolving Conflict. A Practical Approach*, 2nd edition, Oxford University Press, Oxford & New Royk 1999: 6-14.

Weil, S., *The Need for Roots*, Routledge, London & New York, 2003 (original 1949).

Wicclair, M.R., "Ethics, community and the elderly: health care decision-making for incompetent elderly patients", in Michael Parker (ed.) *Ethics and Community in the Health Care Professions*, Routledge, London & New York, 1999: 135-153.

Woodward, K., *Ageing and its Discontents: Freud and Other Fictions*, Indiana University Press, Bloomington and Indianapolis, 1991.

Chapter 8
Biopsychosocial and end-of-life care – timely intervention for elderly[1]

End-of-life decisions are not only about palliation and advanced directives. The biopsychosocial model is a paradigm which helps identify the psychological and social factors and barriers which help towards a realistic balance towards the end-of-life. Spirituality in particular, is not merely religious practices and the presence of pastoral care, but is about achieving balance, harmony and meaning. New models can help for the elderly in extending the concept of palliative care at the very end of terminal diseases to more chronic and disabling conditions which affect the outcome. Moreover one should not consider end-of-life decision based merely on age, but in the case of the elderly palliation and other biopsychosocial decisions which would otherwise be directed only in terminal illness, need to be considered earlier.

There is much to be argued in favour of not confusing end-of-life with mere aging. We usually speak about end-of-life when a typical case as discussed in the beginning of the article presents itself. Even in such circumstances one can postpone end-of-life decisions such as palliative care until such time as is needed 'biologically'. Aspects of the biopsychosocial model, spirituality and healing, and a Timely and Longitudinal (TLC) model are discussed.

The biopsychosocial model

The biopsychosocial (BPS) model had been described as a paradigm in the philosophy of family practice and is quite acceptable in curricula and methodology today (MsWhinney, 1997). However when it comes to end-of-life, there is considerable discussion of 'healing' and other

[1] Mallia, P., "Biopsychosocial and End-of-Life Care – timely intervention for Elderly", *Journal of the International Institute on Aging,* 2010: 20(4); 22-29.

psychosocial issues such as spirituality, that it is quite appropriate to use this paradigm also within the hospital and/or hospice setting. It may also be the case that for the elderly especially the buck stops within the realm of family practice. Of all health care professionals it is the primary care physician who is best situated to assist the elderly patient and is ideally suited to take into consideration intrinsic factors such as illness and extrinsic factors such as family concerns and wishes and indeed the settings of care and financial considerations (Taler & Waymach, 1989). Whilst death is an impending inevitability it is recognized that obtaining consent can be a problem (Rikkert et al., 1996)

The first difficulty in many cases is what amount of information to tell the patient. Families may frequently be against the concept giving bad news to their elderly parents. Whilst this is often a first reaction to protect their loved ones from emotion burden, there are instances where it is entrenched in different ideals. The concept of truth telling has centred around Western ethics, but may vary with different cultures (Crane, M., & Wittink, M., 2005). Searight and Gafford (2005) list four primary reasons for nondisclosure:

- Certain cultures which view discussion of serious illness as disrespectful
- Certain cultures which view open discussion of serious illness as provoking depression or anxiety which the patient can do without
- Cultures which view that disclosure may eliminate hope, and
- Cultures which assert that speaking or alluding to serious illness can indeed bring about death or bring about terminal illness because of the power of the spoken word.

They point out literature that indicates that many Asian cultures, for example, perceive it as unnecessarily cruel to directly inform a patient of a cancer diagnosis, and that even amongst European cultures, such disclosure is disrespectful and inhumane. The authors quote this amongst Bosnian-American and Italian-American immigrants and moreover noticed that Bosnian immigrant doctors 'go around' a diagnosis. When considering truth telling, the Western assertion that many patients actually want to be told the truth, has to be balanced against the harm to health which may be caused by someone who is already suffering pain and now is given an emotional burden. It would be interesting to have a comparative study of attitudes of patients and doctors in different European countries, singling out Europe since it is usually classified as Western when it comes to discussion of ethical values.

The biological

Much end-of-life decisions and discussions have to do with the 'biological', such as Advance Directives and extraordinary treatment. However very few Americans, for example, have Advance Directives (Crane & Wittink, 2005) and it is presumed here that the number decreases in Europe and even more in other continents. It is appropriate therefore to discuss the wishes of the patient in advance and where the patient lacks decision-making capacity, to discuss these issues with family members (Lang & Quill, 2004). The ethical, legal, familial and communication issues are complex. Without legal guidance, Lang and quill note that the most frequent hierarchy used in the United States is the spouse, then the adult children, and then the parents. Of course physicians are guided to encourage the persons acting on behalf of patients to act in their best interests, especially acting upon what the patients would have wished, or what they thought they would have wished. It has been shown that this not only decreases feelings of guilt afterwards should difficult decisions be taken but discourages family members to make decisions based upon their personal values alone (*ibid.*, p. 720).

Lang and Quill recommend that the family are made to appreciate the clinical situation and the prognosis and be prepared to provide support if the expectations are higher than the situation allows. Questions such as "Do you want to have everything done for your (parent)?" should be avoided and everyone would presumably want the best done for a loved one (*ibid.*, p. 721). These should be substituted by a discussion of the differences and expectations of whether everything should be done for *comfort* or for *survival.* Often families feel undecided about feeding and hydration as they fear that the patient is being deprived and induced into feeling thirst or greater distress. It should be helpful to discuss that interest in food decreases towards the end and that medical observation has shown that artificial nutrition often increases the patient's awareness of discomfort and distress rather than allowing one to fall gradually into a coma; therefore stopping of feeding can indeed decrease distress (*ibid.*, p. 721). Discussing 'how to decide' is therefore important to be done before discussing 'what to be done'. One should establish how and by whom decision are to be taken, making it clear that there is also a difference between a 'substituted judgement' and a decision in 'the best interests of the patient'. Substituted judgements can be laden with values of who is making the decision. Lang & Quill also note that it is important to recognize, that when one is faced with an Advance Diretive, a decision not to be put on a respirator or some other form of artificial treatment, may have been referring to a particular circumstance, such as a massive cerebral haemorrhage and may not have meant to apply to all situations.

Many families appreciate their physicians' input and advice and may indeed seem to be relinquishing their autonomy. It should be understood that if the physician has understood and listened to all concerned and has shared his or her opinion, following the physician's recommendation is another form of exercising one's autonomy as, once information and good communication has occurred, it is on a voluntary basis that one *chooses* to act under the influence of someone deemed to be more competent in such choices (Beauchamp & Childress, 1994).

Reichel (1999) points out that family practice as a specialty has a great deal to contribute to end-of-life care and it is strategically placed and indeed family physicians are numerous enough to provide such care. He quotes Byock (1997) who spoke of 'dying well', 'living while dying', and 'physician-assisted living', so as to change our attitudes of death to one of being a time of 'love and reconciliation, and a time of transcendence of suffering'.

The psychosocial

Celler et al. (2004) suggest that a multidisciplinary research study designed to monitor changes in simple measures as mobility, sleep patterns, washing and toilet facilities, utilization of cooking etc can bring abut timely and cost-effective intervention of medical and community-based services. But whilst even family physicians can help dying patients and their families to focus on pain management and increased home care, increased advance directives etc., the frequency of the latter proved unlikely to improve the care of the dying patient and that the support of better communication and more comprehensive health care planning legislative frameworks can help the family physician facilitate this process (Reichel, 1999). In this regard it is interesting to note studies which show that patients desire even spiritual discussions with their physicians and that patients felt that physician inquiry about spirituality or religious beliefs is appropriate. In a study (McCord et al, 2004) to determine the appropriateness of physician enquiry into these areas, and the reasons why patients would wish their physicians to know about their spiritual beliefs and indeed what they would wish for their physicians to do with such information, found that patients do indeed desire these discussion and that 13% up to 73% of patients (from out-patient studies) want physicians to have knowledge of their spiritual or religious beliefs but that these discussion were indeed rare. Amongst the problems which physicians raise for this include departing from traditional medical agendas, lack of spiritual training, and whether it is ethical to have physicians as pastoral counsellors. There is also the possibility of doing harm, time constraints and invasion of privacy issues and in determining which patients would want to talk. The study was intended to help physicians with these issues. It showed, amongst other points, that many patients want this sort of discussion so that:

- The doctor can understand how one's beliefs influence one's decisions
- The doctor can better understand the patient
- The doctor can provide compassion
- The doctor can refer to a spiritual advisor if necessary

The percentage of those welcoming the inquiry increased with the severity of the illness. The authors thus argue that strict scientific approaches overlook the importance of the meaning of life and hope to patients' well-being. They indicate that their sample was overrepreseentative of white population and better educated women. The study also found that those over 60 years were more likely to participate in the study than those between 30-64 years of age, observing that this group were usually significantly sicker, which is why they refused to participate. This may have implications for elderly who are ill and in their management of this problem.

Spirituality in health management?

In a qualitative analysis, Daaleman et al. (2008) concluded that clinicians and other health professionals consider spiritual care at the end-of-life as a series of interpersonal process in the context of human values and experiences, rather than a prescribed role. It is more a recognition of "human value, dignity, and shared decision-making, rather than through shared practice (ie, prayer), or through discussions of religious or theological issues at the bedside." Daaleman and Frey (2004) also tested a useful research tool (the Spirituality Index of Well-Being (SIWB)), and found it to be a valid and reliable instrument, that can be used in health-related quality-of-life studies.

The distinction between spirituality and religiosity is made. Daaleman, Perera and Studenski (2004) found that religious practices are much associated with functional status in the elderly and that "geriatric out-patients who report greater spirituality, but not greater religiosity, are more likely to appraise their health as good". They acknowledge that religion and spirituality are important psychosocial factors in the lives of elderly, but distinguish that religiosity is viewed as the various organized, individual, and attitudes of various religious traditions. These are usually traditional practices. Spirituality is the expression of meaning and purpose (as discussed in this paper). Religious service attendance is significantly associated with functional status which accounts for the variation in reported health status. Elders with greater religiosity were less likely to report good health status than those with greater spirituality. However race, physical functioning and quality of life can all affect religious practice (*ibid.*).

Healing

'Healing' is a word which is much broader than 'cure'; in and of itself includes the spiritual side of the social context of the biopsychosocial. If one focuses on the phase of life when one is elderly as part of an approach towards an end-of-life process, one should perhaps concentrate on a process of 'healing', as there often is no cure for ailments which afflict the elderly population, such as decreased mobility due to arthritis and neurological conditions such as Parkinson's, and cardiac and respiratory condition, etc. If helplessness is one of the unpleasant experiences which induces suffering, this must not be overlooked in the elderly and therefore in the management by physicians and health care workers and their understanding of suffering and healing. Hsu et al. (2008) studied various groups, including patients, nurses and primary care physicians, in focus groups in a qualitative analysis. They found that healing is a multidimensional process which involves physical, emotional and spiritual dimensions. The key 'themes' were that:

- Healing is multidimensional and holistic
- Healing is a process (or a journey)
- The goal of healing is recovery or restoration
- Healing requires the person to reach a personal balance and acceptance
- Relationships are essential to healing.

This implies that if physicians show a lack of capacity for empathy, communication, and relationship, then they are not in a good position to contribute to healing (*ibid.*). The authors understood that their basic assumption that many people would expect healing to come from within the realm of alternative and/or spiritual practices, to be false, implying of course that participation of the healing process is part of the phenomenon and expectation of the doctor-patient relationship.

Hsu et al. (2008) showed that physicians do understand that a lot of the healing process occurs without their intervention. They usually function not as agents but as facilitators. Many people which form meaningful relationships can therefore participate in the process of healing. Also, healing is a dynamic process of recovering from trauma or illness. In this regard, the process is achieved by "working towards realistic goals, restoring function and regaining a personal sense of balance and peace". As facilitators, a key component imparted by clinicians and staff in the clinical setting is a feeling or caring, connection and warmth (*ibid.*).The importance of 'time' was emphasized and that therefore the time the physician or carer spends with the person is essential; whilst patients expressed that it is the quality of time rather than quantity that is important. Professionals' own experiences of healing indeed facilitated the process. Conversely it was simply the absence of positive facilitators that provided the mayor barriers to an effective healing process. A negative encounter even at a front desk was described as having a negative effect on the overall healing process whilst in the clinic setting. However both patients and physicians emphasized that a mayor barrier can be the patients themselves and that they therefore bear the central responsibility for healing.

In the study, few participants spoke of faith healing and divine intervention, but more of a wholeness of mind, body and spirit, notwithstanding that in much literature spirituality is central to the healing process. Also participant focused less on suffering and more on restoration of function, (which can have important implications for the elderly population). In this study participants were mostly white, and spoke about relationships with primary care physicians. They were generally described as being more educated and less religious than in many regions. However the research raises fundamental questions about the goals of health care and medicine.

Conversely, Egnew (2005) interviewed renowned authors in the field of goals of medicine and palliation. These included Eric, J. Cassell, Elisabeth Kubler-Ross, and Dame Cicely Saunders amongst others. In these interviews, the premise was that healing in a holistic sense has faded from medical attention and is rarely discussed in medical literature. Indeed the nursing literature reflects increasing concern with healing and it is pointed out that the fact that medicine has no accepted definition of holistic healing is a 'curiosity', and that if healing is a core function of medicine, then exploration of its symbolic meaning compels more organized research into the phenomenon. The definition of the above three interviewees all included the concept of 'wholeness', whilst others related to a state of mind and other spiritual experiences such as harmony between mind, body and spirit. Egnew notes that the term healing is derived from the root *haelem*, and a condition of being in *hal*, which means wholeness. To heal is therefore to make 'sound or whole', and therefore defining the process of healing as one involving a search for wholeness is indeed well-founded. 'Ill persons undergo transformation in which they are unable to be he persons they once were. This threat to wholeness generates suffering and involves the physical, social, psychological, and spiritual dimension of personhood…Suffering is an inherently unpleasant experience reflecting perception of helplessness'. One cannot help note how this definition would encompass many elderly people who have also underwent this *transformation*.

Timely, longitudinal and collaborative care

Jerant et al. (2004) have identified five fundamental problems with current palliative care, which are discussed briefly here. They write in the context of extending our normal definitions of palliative care for terminal disease and incorporate it in an earlier phase of life, which can thus be adopted for use in the elderly population, who may suffer from chronic and disabling disease. The first problem they identify with current palliative care for elderly is thus that it is considered a terminal event rather than a longitudinal process. This could be an unintended consequence of hospices and hospice movements who defer palliative care to when the patient is expected to die soon. But older patients typically have more chronic and slowly progressive illness with multiple acute episodes, but which nevertheless can cost considerable distress. The result, they argue, is a missed opportunity for the use of palliative care as well as late referrals to hospices. Whilst admitting elderly to hospices at an early stage may not however be the main objective of hospices, the authors are right in not allowing such a term to be the exclusive field of the final stages of a terminal illness. A model for palliation in the elderly can easily be adopted in homes for the elderly and indeed in community care.

The second problem identified is that palliative care is defined within causal and symptom/sign-specific realm. They argue that palliative care is often defined therefore within a 'false dichotomy' of symptom and disease. Whilst it is true that this argument holds to the extent that palliative care starts late in the disease process, it is only arguably true that once it has started, it is. Nevertheless, the *definition* of when to start palliative care is indeed dependent on the disease progress. Extended palliative care to the elderly would thus mean looking beyond such a definition of *when to start* and consider starting earlier. The authors submit that only treatment intend distinguishes palliative care from normal treatment which is usually oriented to saving life and preventing death. In palliative care it is mainly symptom relief and comfort/care which the focus and not so much to extend life. Taking a decision to start this form of care earlier can have considerable quality of life implications for elderly with chronic and disabling conditions. One needs to contend that this is not necessarily strictly true for medical treatment, whilst it is true for the psychosocial element. Take, for example, treating conditions which require increasing use of opioids. In the terminally ill one is not necessarily concerned with addiction and invocation of the principle of double effect is legitimate, i.e. bringing about the death when the intention was intending palliation. Would this be legitimate in treating severely disabling conditions like arthritis or would this be considered a form of euthanasia. One may contend that unless one is to use such strong medicines earlier, then palliative treatment already occurs, for treating arthritis, for example one does not necessarily intend prolongation or saving of life.

Thirdly, the authors argue that the decision to authorize and focus on palliative care is not usually explicitly negotiated but is a decision taken by health care teams. They argue that although there is a tacit negotiation between physicians, patients and family members, the negotiation should be more explicit. They present a linear relationship between the amount of palliative care and time. As time moves along, there is more change of a tacit agreement to shift curative to palliative care. More explicit agreements may shift this linear relationship to the let and bring about choices to negotiate palliation earlier on. Fourthly, it seems to the authors hat when it comes to respecting the autonomy of patients in treatment choices, we tend to concentrate more on curative options; that is, when we are not yet in the palliative stage. Thus, asking patients whether they want invasive and advanced forms of treatment when there is no chance of survival may not be the appropriate approach to elderly either and allowing people to come to terms with their illness trajectory may allow for a better quality of life oriented approach and to a palliative care rather than life-saving care.

Finally, palliative care occurs *outside* the usually processes. There come a point when one decides to stop normal curative treatment and 'shift' to palliative care. The authors suggest a more integrated process for 'palliative care delivery to become and integral part of daily clinical practice, and to facilitate deeper, less hurried, longitudinal palliative care dialogues'. The key here is the *longitudinal* process rather than an immediate (transverse) change from one form of therapy to another.

The TLC (Timely/Team, Longitudinal, & Collaborative/Comprehensive) model which the authors present is based therefore on bringing in palliative care earlier, with an evolving balance (longitudinal) of curative vs palliative and more collaboratively. This model helps significantly with the case discussed in the beginning. If we start with 'collaborative', the concept of truth telling becomes something which the family dialogue can negotiate more effectively rather than seeing truth-telling merely from a Westernized 'rights' approach. This allows for more cultural input, giving this ethical concept a more 'comprehensive' twist. Naturally the 'team' approach would include the family as part of the team but any necessary input on patients' rights and the advantages thereof may be brought in without undue pressure by the physicians themselves. A timelier introduction of palliation of course intends it to be earlier and in good time, whilst at the same time not intending that the transition is directly from a curative to a palliative but a gradual 'longitudinal' one.

Studies are of course necessary to assess outcomes and satisfaction by bringing in palliative care earlier and gradually. There are however good moral arguments from a patient-dignity point of view. Death is not seen as something to fight, and treatment of cancer becomes something to deal with plaintively as well. But it also means that realistic goals are given to family and patients alike accepting the inevitability of death and that 'everything is (being) done' for these goals, rather than for (often unrealistic) goals of trying to cure an illness. Admittedly the latter seems to give the perception of allowing more hope to patients. But we know that such hope is false and deceptive and is given only charitably because of our fears of causing distress. We have seen however that truth telling is something that must be negotiated as well rather than imposed. One does not necessarily need to invoke a right and it is the responsibility of the care-giver to find the weight the patient attaches to this right. Conversely it should be noted that studies do show that, when asked whether palliative care referral was done 'too late' or not, relatives of patients of young patients were less likely to say that referral was 'too late', and moreover respondents of deceased who suffered from chronic condition such as obstructive lung disease as well as respondents with higher education were more likely to believe that the hospice referral was late as well (Williams, 2008). It is also recognized that most specialties are treating an increasing number of elderly and that there are managements decisions beyond simple diagnosis and treatment to make the ethical and legal issues of elderly very important (Vassallo, 2004), especially in the management of dementia.

Conversely timely discussion with relatives can bring about less stress to the carers. Robinson and Thurnher (1979) had shown that deterioration in family relationships ca begin early especially with a parent's mental impairment. Providing adult children with better awareness of mental impairment circumvents this problem. Confinement of the adult children also contributed to stress. Confinement can mean also the infringement on life-style which the care of the parent brings about. A comprehensive approach would contribute to a better understanding of how the illness/aged person interacts with the family to bring about better outcomes in choice of (timely) available resources.

Conclusion

There is much to be argued in favour of not confusing end-of-life with mere aging. We usually speak about end-of-life when a typical case as discussed in the beginning of the article presents itself. Even in such circumstances one can postpone end-of-life decisions such as palliative care until such time as is needed 'biologically'. One needs to ask how such models affect the case scenarios; for if one is to change a paradigm of action, it will need to be considered in every case.

Physicians are not trained to hear stories and narratives and often fail to elicit many of the patient's non-medical concerns. Indeed many question the legitimacy of the physicians' role as being guides for patients. Yet changes in medicine are reflecting a progress in addressing holistic approaches and a shift of incorporating care into cure, if indeed to cure is also to care. Whilst for many physicians an illness may be a routine incident in a daily round, to the patient it is a crises in life; for many a crises of meaning. To help patients transcend this suffering in the realm of old age, a metamorphosis of a doctor from a 'doer to helper' and from an expert problem solver and fixer to a companion (Egnew, 2009) is necessary in the bag of clinical skills needed to manage a growing population of chronically ill patients, many of whom are indeed our elderly population. A shift in the timing, administration and comprehensiveness of palliative care plus a participation in the psychosocial aspects and importance of wholeness and healing can have improved outcomes on end-of-life approaches to the elderly population. Certainly this may fit well into the philosophy of family medicine.

References

Byock I, *Dying well: the prospect for growth at the need of life*. New York: Riverhead, 1992.

Celler BG, Remote monitoring of health status of the elderly at home. A multidisciplinary project on aging at the University of New South Wales, *International Journal of Bio-Medical Computing*, 1995; 40(2): 147-155.

Crane MC, Doukas DJ, Respecting End-of-Life Treatment Preferences, *American Family Physician*, 2005; 72:1263-1270.

Daaleman TP, Frey BB, Spirituality Index of Well-Being: A New Instrument for health-Related Quality-of-Life Research, *Annals of Family Practice*, 2(5), September/October 2004: 499-503.

Daaleman TP, Perera S, Studenski SA, Religion, Spirituality, and Health Status in Geriatric Outpatients, *Annals of Family Medicine*, 2(1), January/February 2004: 49-53.

Daaleman TP, Ushe BM, Williams SW, Rawlings,J, Hanson LC. An Exploratory Study of Spiritual Care at the End-of-life, *Annals of Family Practice*, 6(5), September/October 2008: 406-411.

Egnew TR. Suffering, Meaning, and Healing: Challenges of Contemporary Medicine, *Annals of Family Medicine*, 7(2), March/April 2009: 170-175.

Egnew TR. The Meaning of Healing: Transcending Suffering, *Annals of Family Medicine*¸ 3(3), May/June 2005: 255-262.

Hsu C, Phillips WR, Sherman KJ, Hawkes R, Cherkin DC. Healing in Primary Care: A Vision Shared by Paients, Physicians, Nurses, and Clinical Staff, *Annals of Family Medicine*, 6(4), July/August 2008: 307-314.

Jerant AF, Azari RS, Nesbitt TS, Meyers FJ, The TLC Model of Palliative Care in the Elderly: Preliminary Application in the Assisted Living Setting, *Annals of Family Medicine*, 2(1), January/February 2004: 54-60.

Lang F, Quill T. Making Decisions with Families at the End-of-life, *American Family Physician* 2004; 70: 719-726.

McCord G, Gilchrist VJ, Grossman SD, King BD, McCormick KF, Oprandi AM, Schrop SL, Selius BA, Smucker WD, Weldy DL, Amorn M, Carter MA, Deak AJ, Hefzy H, Srivastava M. Discussing Spirituality With Patients: A Rational and ethical Approach, *Annals of Family Practice*, 2(4), July/August 2004: 356-361.

McWhinney IR. *A Textbook of Family Medicine*, 2nd ed. Oxford University Press, New York, 1997.

Olde Rickert MGM, Ten Have H., Hoefnagels W. Informed consent in biomedical studies on aging: survey of four journals, *BMJ*, 1996; 313:1117.

Reichel W. End-ofLife Care and Family Practice, Editorial, *American Family Physician,* March 15, 1999.

Robinson B, Thurnher M. Taking Care of Aged Parents: A Family Cycle Transition, *the Gerontologist*, 1979; 19(6): 566-593.

Searight HR, Gafford J. Cultural Diversity at the End-of-life: Issues and Guidelines for Family Physicians, *American Family Physician*, 71(3), February 1, 2005: 515-522.

Taler GA, Waymakc MH. Ethics and the elderly, *Primary Care*, 1989; 16(2): 529-541.

Vassallo M, book review, Medical Ethics and the Elderly, *Journal of the Royal Society of Medicine*, 2004: 97(9): 454

Williams ME, Ensminger WK, Williams ME. Ethics and Quality of life in the Elderly: Recent Advances, *highlights of the American Geriatrics Society*, 2008: http://cme.medscape.com/viewarticles/577607.

Chapter 9
Palliative sedation and removal of artificial nutrition and hydration at the end-of-life[1]

Recently considerable concern has been expressed, especially in religious circle, on whether palliative sedation is a form of euthanasia. Palliative sedation is intended as a form of palliative care when there is intractable pain, that is, pain which is not removed by normal means of medication. The controversy is not sedation per se, but sedation to unconsciousness with the intent of allowing the patient to die in that state. This paper discusses the issue of palliative sedation, referring especially to inherent problems such as removal of hydration and feeding, and whether it is licit for existential suffering, but also its use in environments outside hospital settings, such as home care.

Concerns and issues

There are conflicting views about the morality of palliative sedation, but it would seem that most studies show that palliative sedation (PS) does not shorten the life of the individual. Murray and Jennings (2000) say that "our approach to end-of-life decision-making has been excessively rationalistic, arguing that many do not plan ahead and even those who do may find it difficult to implement. Moreover attitudes towards future planning and control do not seem to travel well across cultures". However the Catholic culture remains one that even within itself continues to pose problems on end-of-life for many. Controversies exist and some have argued that prolonging life indefinitely is perverse; but that not all Catholics think this way (Dugdale & Ridenour, 2011). Indeed one cannot but wonder whether recent decades of bioethics and media coverage of hot cases has led to a more confused approach

[1] Mallia, P., "On the licitness of inducing Palliative Sedation and removal of Artificial Nutrition and Hydration at the End-of-life", *International Journal of Bioethics*, 2014, 24(2): 67-82

to death. At least as far back as the sixties there was no controversy on allowing people to die, which even meant removing feeding and hydration. Pius XII's (Pope) allocutions seem to be clouded nowadays, especially with advancing medical practice. Hinton (1967) referring to Pius XII's work stated that "It breaks no unalterable Christian law, if, on the principle of loving his neighbour as himself, a doctor allows a person to die". Pius XII's decision was already preceded by many moral positions that it should not be obligatory to take extraordinary measures at the end-of-life. What these statements, which now find themselves worded in the Catholic Catechism, made clear was that there was no need to be scrupulous with *under-treating* a patient at the end-of-life. Conversely, by double effect a doctor, following a standard of care, may indeed *increase* doses of pain relief even if these can be the final cause of death. Naturally one would not expect that a doctors jump to give a high doses immediately; standard pathways for increasing doses (such as the step-up and step-down systems) exist. This position was taken recently by the International Association of Catholic Bioethicist (2011). However their position remains unclear whether existential suffering alone can constitute a legitimate claim for sedation. This not so much because it hastens death, something which many seem to agree that it does not, but because it may deprive the person of last moments reconciliation and preparation for death.

Invariably there comes a time when pain relief may bring about sedation; but should it deliberately be sought? Morphine, for example, can also sedate a patient, but this is a side-effect of its use for relieving pain. Nevertheless, that side-effect had its inherent benefits.

The controversy is whether one should use these inherent beneficial side-effects as an ultimate goal to reduce not only pain but emotional and existential pain assuming that the intention is always, as was for palliative relief, considered charitable towards the patient and not to bring about an earlier death or euthanasia.

Whilst it is important to acknowledge that parties may disagree and that some have tackled the question of whether PS is slow euthanasia (van Delden, 2007; Hartocollis, 2009) others take an opposing view (Baumann, Claudot, Audibert, Mertes and Puybasset, 2011; O'Reilly, 2008; Simon, Kar, Hinz, & Beck, 2007). There is also literature which compares the two positions (Csikai, 1999; Rietjens, et al., 2006;

Krishna, 2011). Palliative sedation has been shown that it can safely be offered at home too (Science Daily, 2010).

In this regard the Liverpool Pathway (2010), used in the UK at the end-of-life has been criticized lately by a Maltese physician working in the UK (Doughty, 2012), saying that this pathway is tantamount to euthanasia. Prof. Saunders, who is chairman of the Royal College of Physicians of London's Ethics committee, who is known not to favour euthanasia, has criticized this view and said that the Liverpool Pathway not only does not cause euthanasia but has helped a lot of people die a peaceful death (*ibid.*). Before its introduction it was considered that only 16% of patients dying of cancer received such care in the hospice setting. The idea was to transfer what was being done in hospices to general hospitals. Hospices were originally pioneered by Dame Cicely Saunders, who was esteemed in this regard and never accused of any form of euthanasia. In fact she was a staunch opponent of euthanasia and Admiraal, a Dutch physician who advocates euthanasia, had accused hospices of giving 'cocktails' to people to sedate them (Dunnett, 1999). So the question inevitably is why should such care, transferred to a general hospital provide controversy? Whether and when a person is put on the pathway is a clinical decision taken by both patient and doctor. The UK has had many contestations, such as the case of Diane Pretty, where people wanted assistance with removal of life-support measures. The law against euthanasia was always upheld and one cannot doubt the countries' stance in this regard. Yet the Department of Health has recommended the LCP as the best practice model for end-of-life and the Catholic Herald (2010) condoned it if used appropriately. At the end of the day, like with any application of the principle of double effect, the agent must intend only the good, and therefore the pathway is dependent on the moral agent. Any criticism must go to those who use the pathway inappropriately.

One contending matter in the LCP is whether existential suffering is a form of legitimate pain/suffering. It is usually accepted that palliative pain relief, by double effect, can be given even in the knowledge that it can inadvertently cause the death of the individual, so long as this is foreseen but unintended. However, this usually applies to suffering from pain; what is questioned is existential suffering. Another question is the removal of hydration and nutrition when appropriate; the

American Journal of Hospice and Palliative Care (Craig, 2005) has criticized the LCP in this regard for not taking an explicit position. This, in fact seem to be a good thing, as removal of AHN should not be deliberate but dependent upon the situation. Although doctors had criticized this pathway, it would seem that this resulted from lack of awareness and knowledge in the use of the pathway, as the Association for Palliative Medicine and the anti-euthanasia charity (Care Not Killing) called this criticism inaccurate (Association for Palliative Medicine, 2009). No studies to prove that the LCP is abused or being used early have however been produced.

The ethical questions to sedation to unconsciousness and the removal of ANH can be viewed in the light of the much-lauded biopsychosocial model used in palliative care, the question of the difference in standards of care between home- and hospital- care, and even a questioning of the legitimacy to speak about 'existential' suffering in the face of treatment.

Biopsychosocial approach to existential pain

The biopsychosocial (BPS) approach to health care has recognized that one cannot objectify suffering by reducing it solely to its biological causes. It recognizes that a holistic approach to health care must take into consideration the psychological and social aspects, the latter including religious (and therefore also called bio-psycho-social-religious). The BPS model has become also a paradigm of primary care (McWhinney, 2009) and has also become standard practice in medicine and nursing in general. Indeed physiotherapy and occupational therapy have always looked at this aspect of care. Emergency situations may not always necessitate the early introduction of the model but it may become necessary during recovery from surgery or other acute conditions.

Is existential pain, pain or suffering? Is it legitimate to be considered within a BPS approach to care? There is considerable overlap between suffering and pain. It is unlikely that guidelines, such as the Catholic teaching on palliative treatment of pain, actually distinguish between pain and suffering. One can be in a lot of pain but not actually 'suffer' from it. Indeed one may welcome the pain from a spiritual point of view. But this cannot apply to everyone. Conversely one may not have actual physical pain but have an emotional suffering of the fact that she is going to die. Palliative care adopts this model of caring as a holistic approach to the dying.

Three arguments seem to be pertinent. The argument that palliative sedation is not a solution for existential suffering seems to have mostly a religious taste. It can be argued that this stage in life can be important for the person to come to terms with death and perhaps even reconcile with God. Does this argument presume that the person has *not* done his reconciliations? The question then becomes whether we ought to make such an assertion and allow people to suffer for it. It seems that this sort of reasoning invades the person's right to die a peaceful death because we are preoccupied with 'saving a soul'. Even if this is the case it is too presumptuous to think that God will judge a person at that stage of life; moreover, one is forced to question any validity of reconciliations when one is loaded with medication. Harsh as this may sound, it prevents us from inducing undue suffering in a dying patient who needs our care. Whilst there is no doubt that religious counselling and help in these last stages are important for those who want them, or at least offered to those who come from certain faiths, whether they can be imposed as a policy and deprive sedation is dubious.

The second argument asks what is wrong with unconsciousness itself. There are many situations in life where it is acceptable to be unconscious. There is decreased consciousness even with alcohol, which for many people is a ritual. This leads to unconsciousness in many instances. As long as the person is not a danger to others, there can be no reason to outlaw this. One may question the morality of drinking to this extent; but it is still a free choice. More importantly we accept temporary unconsciousness in many health care situations, surgery being the most common. Even hypnosis is a state of mind (and altered consciousness) which can be induced into a state of forgetfulness such that after the hypnotic session the patient forgets what went on. Unconsciousness in surgery is the same – under anaesthesia, amnesiacs are given so that any undue experience is forgotten. The controversy is whether it is legitimate at the end-of-life. In and of itself therefore 'unconsciousness' is not a wrong; it is bringing it during a controversial time which is questioned. If the intention is to sedate, and sedation in itself is a good, can one consider the timing at end-of-life a foreseen but *unintended* harm, and therefore legitimately follow double effect? When existential pain and suffering cannot be relieved should we persist in delaying or negating this form of treatment on religious grounds?

Thirdly we must seriously question whether the issue of existential suffering should be considered appropriate once the patient is already on a cocktail of medications which can in themselves alter conscious states.

Standard of care, negligence, and double effect

To answer these questions more properly however, one must first consider the conjuring of double effect within the scope of negligence, which is often ignored in philosophical debates of this nature. Double effect recognizes that a bad may be done in trying to bring about a good. It follows that if the four conditions of double effect are fulfilled, then it should be permissible. The condition that 'the bad must not be the means of bring about the good', and therefore that the bad must be indirect, is key to this argument. Granted that if the intention is not to kill the patient (and that therefore the moral agent must intend only the good), the main question is whether unconsciousness at the end-of-life can ever be a good or whether it may be viewed as an unintended harm.

If one were not to be over scrupulous one has to concede that sedation must sometimes be necessary to relief suffering. But given that existential pain is, biologically defined, not a physical pain as that caused by the pathology, it can only be described as existential *suffering*. But to separate *suffering* from physical pain deceives the end of the BPS suffering; it is merely a departure from a standard of care which has become acceptable and indeed required, especially in palliative care. What this means is that suffering has to be seen as something which should be alleviated as well. If we cannot alleviate it by other means then we should consider sedation; titrated and up to unconsciousness if necessary – the unintended harm. Sedation does not come about deliberately but as a consequence of a necessity to titrate higher to achieve proper relief.

It is here that negligence takes an important role; a role which should alleviate fears of deliberately shortening life. Negligence is based, according to tort law, on four conditions: there is a professional duty; there is a departure from that professional duty; a harm is caused; there has to be a connection (nexus) between the harm and the departure from the professional duty. Now professional duty is defined by a standard of care. This is also explored below in the context of palliative sedation in primary care. For the time being we need a standard of care as a professional duty from which to depart for us to define a malpractice. Once harm is caused we speak about negligence. The harm can be thought of as a deliberate hastening of death or a careless administration of a treatment which could otherwise have been avoided. Although it may be difficult to prove, inquiry can show any departures from standards of care when looking at treatment charts, schedules, timing of decisions, what was put down in the notes, and, if necessary, even post mortem toxicology tests. However it may be difficult to define the intentions of 'the moral agent'; but this is the case even with normal palliative treatment under double effect.

A deliberate intention of offering permanent sedation without trying to alleviate suffering omits the paradigm of the BPS approach ad as well is perhaps a harm even if it does not bring about death. Agreeing with terminally ill patients that they can choose to be immediately sedated when they enter hospital for the final time should probably be considered wrong if it is merely used to avoid a difficult situation without considering whether the person may live that situation without undue suffering. However it would constitute a departure from a standard of care *not* to discuss it as an option of last resort early on in planning care. Patients may be restricted from 'requesting' it without due consideration and counselling insofar as they cannot request things which are not standards of care. This is understood by noting that even countries which legitimize euthanasia have conditions to be fulfilled to consider the practice a normal standard of care. So, it would be inconceivable that palliative sedation does not have such conditions as well, one of which, for example, would be the failed attempt to alleviate all three of the biological, psychological and social aspects of care.

Standards in primary care

But there remains the fact that standards of care can vary from one specialty to another and from one country to another. In many places in the United States and the United Kingdom, for example, general practitioners would refer terminally ill patients to hospices or hospitals. Here standards of care will vary from those places where 'the buck stops' at home and the patient has to be taken care of in his or her own dwelling. As with Bolam (Howard & Bogle, 2005) one cannot expect that the primary care physician has all the means and equipment at her disposal as the physician in a hospital or hospice setting. Hospital protocols and pathways similar to the LCP may not be feasible or available in certain rural areas or even when patients wish to die at home. Conversely a person wishing to die at home may perceive transfer to hospice or hospital as disproportionate to his or her wishes.

Dying at home has always been known not to bring to the bed side the facilities available in hospital and doctors naturally explain this. Patients understand, but dying at home is part of a holistic care - one passes away in one's environment, in one's own bed, surrounded by one's own family. Does it make a difference having a drip to hydrate someone in the final hours? There is a standard of care to be expected from each specialty and although these may not be as stringent in the home setting for the general practitioner as they would be in the hospital session for a specialized physician, there would still need to be guidelines. However it has to be acknowledged that unless the national health service provides training and tools and unless referral to hospital (providing it is the wish of the patient) is available the situation in primary care is so different as to render the 'existential suffering' argument very dubious.

Is the existential argument always a licit one?

Clearly even a small amount of sedation changes the mental state of the patient. If one drinks a measure of alcohol one may feel better. People are known to drink a small amount of alcohol to 'loosen up' socially. We do not accept driving under the effects of alcohol because we know that even small amounts may change the mental state of a person, which may make him or her, under-cautious and cause harm in the process. Alcohol is known, for example, to decrease the rate of response to a situation.

The same effect can be brought about by any form of sedation or pain relief. Therefore when we speak about 'existential suffering' we are already speaking about a patient who is under the influence of drugs. These certainly affect a controlling influence on any voluntary choice. We cannot assume that once the patient is speaking to us, there can be no side effects of the drug which would make a patient choose something which otherwise she would not have chosen. Under the influence of a pain killer one may feel an attraction to a person which otherwise is not felt. Even normal care produces 'transference' – affective feelings of the patient towards the carer. Once we are dealing with these dire situations it becomes questionable whether we should be speaking of 'existentialism' at all. Even existential suffering may be the result of high doses of pain relief (just as morphine can produce hallucinations, it is not unreasonable to consider existential suffering in this light as well). Does this mean we should remove the pain relief? If the answer is no, which invariably it should be, then one has to put into question any existential suffering and allow space for attributing it to medication and other factors. One should therefore question the reasons why we want people to withstand existential suffering and ask whether it is patient- or carer- centred. Any assumption that they can come to terms with something on a spiritual level cannot be taken for granted as any amount of previous pain relief may put into question any 'coming of terms'.

What this in effect means is that we should not be over-cautious. If one of our patients suddenly feels anger at God, we may not be allowing for the fact that this may not indeed be existential suffering but may be medically induced. At the end of the day, even if they are genuine feelings, we probably should not make value-judgements but be compassionate towards different reactions to facing death, avoiding a verdict to stop treatment short of sedation. Our own spiritual beliefs must be charitable to strengthen rather than hinder us in this regard.

The phenomenon of the doctor patient relationship

The doctor patient relationship does not simply 'happen'. Whilst we speak of principles of beneficence, Nonmaleficence, justice and respect for autonomy, it has been argued that these should be seen through the nature of the doctor patient relationship (Mallia, 2012). Thus the strength of virtues, such as compassion and understanding, fortitude, etc may actually enhance the autonomy of patients to make better choices. Phenomenologically beneficence is the phenomenon of the health care relationship (a phenomenon defined here as that which defines itself in itself), whilst the principle of non-maleficence, is a manifestation of that phenomenon, notwithstanding the term 'primum', in *primum non nocere*. First do not harm does not mean that the intent of beneficence did not come a priori; it is simply a warning that before you act on your good intentions, see that you are following good practice. As discussed, the principle of double effect with regard to palliative care was made to simplify things and to be charitable towards suffering patients. It was made to reassure doctors that treatment, even if it is the cause of death, so long as it is foreseen but unintended, is licit.

The main issue of double effect in palliate care is to help doctors treat patients and to avoid them being scrupulous at an end-of-life situation with consequences for the patient. Some form of sedation most often occurs; what we have now is a situation to make it better. Dying people do not drink and feed; therefore removing these at the very final stages may in fact be a good thing as over-scrupulous ANH can make death itself more burdensome. Again we have to consider people dying at home whose doctors have no access to artificial nutrition and hydration. If this is acceptable then one must question why people at hospital should be made to undergo consequential treatment, including AHN, when at home they would not have received it? After all we do not really know that AHN always improves quality of death; it is an educated guess; believed to bring about comfort. It was not used several decades ago when '*TLC*' – tender loving care – was put on the charts and all treatment and drips removed. For all we know it may deprive, in the last hours or days, a natural death which may be more comfortable.

Unless the doctrine of double effect is to be victim of its own success, palliative sedation should be allowed with specific guidelines and codes of practice. Just as in palliative treatment of biological pain, it is not good practice to jump from a small dose of morphine-like substances to higher doses, but must be titrated; the same goes for palliative sedation. And just as one limits standards of care to the specialty and the situation (one cannot expect the same level of technology at the bedside of a home-dying patient, once informed consent in this regard has been obtained) with titrating doses and which treatments are available, it follows that with hydration, nutrition and sedation, one should reason in the same way. Certainly in the primary care setting of many countries ANH is foreseen although unintended. One can therefore question whether it is always licit in the hospital setting.

Towards a palliative ontology in health care

Within palliative care it is appropriate to reflect more here on the religious aspect, as this is where most of the concern lies. In fact current (Trinitarian) ontology applied to developments in social understanding, including health care gives much importance to decision-making to the quality of the relationship with patients (Cambon, 1999). Arriving to sedation should be seen in the light of the doctor-centred approach; allowing for the relationship and circumstance to act as a guide gives scope for a patient centre approach. Questions of an existential nature should transcend themselves into the nature of a relationship with *this* patient. Sedation has to be seen as an existential choice understood from within the relationship: Trinitarian ontology encourages this 'rapport' as testimony (Caretta, 2007). In this testimony we recall the good Samaritan, who, seeing the injured person was moved and gave him help; covered his wounds; used the oil and *wine* at his disposal; carried him; took him to a hotel; cared for him; paid for him... the sick are a special reality which reflect the cross (Lubich 1997 in Caretta, 2007). Incidentally wine was used to reduce consciousness to lessen the pain up to the modern era.

The objective of health care systems should be to satisfy in the best way the needs and expectations of patients; to give care of the highest quality. The danger of reducing the doctor-patient relationship to technology and therapeutic protocols for diagnosis and treatment – a risk of curing the pathology rather than the person – continues to exist. 'Relationship' means a 'rapport' with the patient, not seen any more from an interventionist point of view, but *with* a person for whom this technology or treatment collaborates *to* the relationship. Since questions of existentialism arise mostly within the religious context, it is appropriate to consider these recent developments in Trinitarian ontology as applied to the doctor/health care provider – patient relationships.

'To really help a person one has to help the sick person feel the attention and interest – element of good communication. This communication requires a true dialogue that 'lives' between giving information and listening; sometimes even seeking a 'language' to communicate with those who cannot due to their disabilities. This attention underlines the uniqueness of each sick person and translates into unique needs and health care 'answers' – even spiritual (Caretta 2007, *ibid*). One notes that sometimes the message of faith is given in a wrong way – by presenting it as some sort of 'placebo' or a 'resource' which is worth using. The proclamation of God's kingdom has to start therefore with our attitudes and relationships (Caretta & Petrini, 1995, p. 77)

Conclusion

The licit-ness of existential suffering has been pointed out in the context of a patient already sedated; a situation which can render persons vulnerable to their own feelings. The fact that ANH is not always given in the context of primary (home) care questions whether this can licitly be imposed in a hospital setting, and, moreover, whereas a different standard of care may be licit in the former setting when palliative relief is given leads us also to question how stringent we should be when people are in a secondary setting when it comes to increasing doses leading to sedation. In this context one can legitimately invoke the doctrine of double effect in which the good is not brought about by a deliberate induction of the harm (sedation and removal of ANH) once this is arrived to consequentially and prudently.

Whilst sedation should therefore probably not be deliberate but seen as a consequential and perhaps unintended arrival point, it must also be seen in its broader context. There is a point where science, philosophy and theology must meet (Piero Coda, 2000). We must perhaps follow developments in this area of ontological enquiry. If there is an area which has commanded the exhaustion of science, philosophy and theology, it is medicine; where biology, technology, ethics, metaphysics and spirituality all converge into the reality of the relationship. The fiduciary bases of the doctor-patient relationship has somewhat been undermined and cannot be taken for granted. The good that respect for autonomy can bring may even isolate the patient and leans us toward a triangulation of provider-patient-rights. We need to shift this triangulation to provider-patient-relationship again. This can only be done by focusing on the communication aspect of the relationship which does not use solely technology as its means but the phenomenon of what makes human nature and understanding itself. This is not merely 'pastoral' care. It is something which health care providers, especially those working in Catholic hospitals (or at least) must develop and cultivate. It helps them grow; doctors *become* doctors in a process of caring. Nurses *become* nurses in a process of caring and serving, etc. It is here that the clinical ethicist plays an important role as clinician/philosopher and who is part of the team fostering this growth.

References

(2010) "A dependable pathway to the life beyond", *Catholic Herald*, 23rd April.

5th IACB International Colloquium, St Charles Borromeo Seminary, Philadelphia, U.S.A., July 10-14, 2011. Topic: Palliative Sedation.

Association for Palliative Medicine. (2009). Liverpool Care Pathway, *Care Not Killing* 15 September.

Baumann, A., Claudot, F., Audibert, G., Mertes, P., and Puybasset, L. (8 February 2011). The ethical and legal aspects of palliative sedation in severely brain-injured patients: A French perspective.

Cambon, E. (1999). *Tinita'. Modello sociale*. Rome: Citta' Nuova Editrice.

Caretta, F. (2007). Sviluppo delle competenze relazionali e qualita' dell'assistenza: il valore aggiunto in sanita'. *Nuova umanita' rivista bimestrale di cultura,* 1(XXIX), 77-89.

Caretta, F., and Petrini, M. (1995). *Accanto al malato lineamenti di assistenza e pastorale*. Italia, Roma: Citta Nuova.

Coda, P. (2000). L'interpretazione del reale. *L'Interpretazione Del Reale; Teologia, Filosofia e Scienza in Dialogo,* 17.

Craig, G. (2008). "Palliative care in overdrive: patients in danger". *Am J Hosp Palliat Care* 25 (2): 155–60.

Csikai, E. L. (1999). Euthanasia and assisted suicide. *Journal of Gerontological Social Work, 31*(3), 49-63.

Doughty, S. (2012). Top doctor's chilling claim: The NHS kills off 130,000 elderly patients every years, Mail Online, 21st June.

Dugdale, L., and Ridenour, A. (2011). Making sense of the roman catholic directive to extend life indefinitely. *The Hastings Centre Report, should Patients always Receive Hard Data about Medical Outcomes?, 41*(2).

Dunnet, A. (1999). *Euthanasia. The heart of the matter*. Hodder & Stoughton, London, Sydney, Auckland, p. 128.

Hartocollis, A. (December 26, 2009). *Hard choice for a comfortable death: Sedation.* Retrieved from http://www.nytimes.com/2009/12/27/health/27sedation.html?pagewanted=1&_r=1

Hinton, J. (1967). *Dying* Penguin Books.

Howard, P., & Bogle. (2005). *Medical law and ethics*. Blackwell Publishing. USA, UK, Australia.

Information for Healthcare Professionals, LCP Central Team. (2010). LCP Central TeamLiverpool Care Pathway for the Dying Patient (LCP), Marie Curie Palliative Care Institute, Liverpool.

Krishna, I., B. C. (2011). Opioid use at the end-of-life: Working out the physician's intentions. *Indian Journal of Medical Ethics,* 8(1).

Mallia, P. (2012). In Ten Have H. (Ed.), *The nature of the doctor-patient relationship. health care principles through the phenomenology of relationships with patients* (1st ed.). USA: Springer.

McWhinney, I. (1989). *A Textbook of Family Medicine*, Oxford University Press, Oxford, New York.

Murray, T. H., and Jennings, B. (2000). The quest to reform end-of-life care: Rethinking assumption and setting new directions. *Improving End-of-life Care,* 52.

O'Reilly, K. (2008). AMA meeting: AMA OKs palliative sedation for terminally ill. *American Medical News, July, 7.*

Rietjens, J., van Delden, J., van der Heide, A., Vrakking, A., Onwuteaka-Philipsen, B., van der Maas, P., & van der Wal, G. (2006). Terminal sedation and euthanasia; a comparison of clinical practices. *American Medical Association.*

Science Daily. (Mar. 2, 2010). Home palliative sedation checklist may ease concerns.

Simon, A., Kar, M., Hinz, J., & Beck, D. (2007). Attitudes towards terminal sedation: An empirical survey among experts in the field of medical ethics. *BMC Palliative Care,* 6, 4. doi: 10.1186/1472-684X-6-4

van Delden, J. J. M. (2007). Terminal sedation: Source of a restless ethical debate. *Journal of Medical Ethics, 33*(4), 187.

Chapter 10
Pathway towards advanced care planning[1]

Introduction

"Death is not primarily a medical event. Death is a personal, relational, and spiritual event, yet the majority of professional effort is concerned with the medical aspects of the end-of-life, often to the neglect of the more pertinent issues facing the dying and their families."[2]

An Advanced Care Plan (ACP) is really a tool using established principles such as the right to refuse treatment at the end-of-life and helping patients and carers approach the end-of-life in a more biopsychosocial manner. As the statement above shows, and there is abundant literature even in medical journals to support this, end-of-life has been only too medicalised. Advanced care plans are an essential component of end-of-life care which often is not considered or is done partially and by different people with little effective and efficient communication. When we decide that the time has come for a patient with ALS to be put on a respirator, the patient can be frowned upon if he or she refuses, as this will lead to immediate death. Yet it is a natural death, and although the treatment will be life-prolonging, as is chemotherapy, the imminence of death puts professionals into a confusion of whether this is morally, legally and medically sound.

Planning in advance helps these decisions. Advance care plan always move according to established laws. They do not of course allow something which is unlawful. Recognizing the imminence of death from as much as a year before to the few days before death allows one to make decisions in good time. Not only medical decisions

---

[1] Mallia, P. (2016) "Pathway Towards Advanced Care Planning" in Pierre Mallia (ed.) *EndCare: An Erasmus+ Project on harmonisation of end-of-life care.* University of Malta.
[2] Watson, M. (2010) "Spiritual Aspects of Advance Care Planning" in K. Thomas and B. Lobo (eds.) *Advance Care Planning in End-of-life Care.* Oxford: Oxford University Press.

are important for patients. One needs time to consider whether they would wish to die at home, and whether there are things to be done which can make their final days better and more bearable. Financial issues can affect decisions, but it is obviously better to consider options in good time than allow to the end.

Often we do not use in good time even the resources we have available. A patient of mine survived breast cancer for ten years. Suddenly it turned worse. There was time to make decisions – an important one would have been to introduce her to hospice. Yet because we sometimes 'fight' cancer we end by not allowing people to appreciate the true situation. This is false hope. This patient suddenly changed for the worse. Her death was even recognised that it would occur within a few days. On a Friday there was a bed crisis and she was sent home to die. Her husband was distraught. She seemed to have been abandoned in the last moments. A discussion with the consultant helped reveal the difficulty he had when it came to admitting more needy patients. But there was also an issue of the fidelity we owe our patients. We are treating individuals and not groups, as is often perceived. It is for this reason that the post Liverpool care pathways document was named *One chance to get it right*. With each patient we only have one chance. If one knows there are bed problems is it even more imperative to have ACPs in place. This patient could have been discharged home with hospice care; her wishes whether to die at home or in hospital could have been known. This can happen even if death is not imminent. Patients with cancer ought to have an opportunity at one stage to discuss what they wish if things start going south.

An ACP ensures that patient's wishes are respected. In the above case it would not have been until the following Monday that the hospice would have been able to see her on such short notice. What will happen in between? What, as expected, she would have died? It would have been a true case of abandonment had the consultant not made the right decision to keep her in hospital after due consideration.

An ACP allows one to make effective use of the team of people we have at our disposal from medics and paramedics, hospice, social services etc. ACP conversation are *voluntary. The National End-of-life Care progamme, UK (2012)* acknowledges that it may be difficult:

> "It is important to remember that ACO conversations are voluntary and whilst some of these conversations may be difficult, they are in fact conversations, which assist and can empower the individual. The conversations can help ensure that individuals retain some control, and that it is their own wishes and preferences that remain the focus of care planning."[3]

The programme uses the acronym ADSE: Ask, Document, Share, Evaluate.[4]

Ask refers to the needs for all those involved in a person's care to ensure the individual is asked and enabled to express their wishes and preferences.

Document refers to the importance of recording the person's wishes and preferences using a standard tool, such as the Preferred Priorities for Care (PPC). Essentially, an individual's wishes can be documented in any form; however, using a tool facilities comprehensive coverage of specific aspects of care and the wishes of the person. It also enables doctors, other professionals and those in close relationships with the person to know clearly what the person's wishes are.

Share refers to the need to have a system in place so that, with the person's consent, their identified wishes and preferences can be shared with all services supporting them.

Evaluate refers to a mechanism by which the impact and effectiveness of using ACPs can be seen within a locality. Evaluation promotes training and understanding to increase effeteness in the facilitation of identifying and supporting individuals' choices and preferences.

There is one caveat which professionals who are versant in some literature ought to be aware of. An ACP is NOT an Advance Directive (AD). Unfortunately many continue to confuse the two. An ACP does not require legislation whilst and AD does. An AD can be done even before a patient is ill and can be done only with a power of attorney and a solicitor or notary. An ACP begins when the person is diagnosed. There is nothing new or illegal than what was done or could have been done before. It is simply a recognition that a model is needed to coordinate the biological, psychological, social and spiritual care of

[3] Pathways through care at the end-of-life. Hayes. A. et al. JKP press 2014.
[4] *ibid.* p. 47.

a person at the end of his or her life. In this there *is* only one chance to get it right with an individual. Failing this we will be failing the patient.

Not coordinating end-of-life care will continue to medicalize care, albeit providing good biological care, but certainly not an ideal in which one may wish to die without extraordinary treatment, or to die at home, and be denied decisions in participating in their care. This leads to debates about euthanasia – something which should be seen a failure of society transforming end-of-life into an abusive non-profit system industry within a hospital system. Abusive because people may easily dump their relatives in hospital because they do not wish to take on the responsibility to help someone who is dying. Secondly because they are not helped in knowing what services are available.

Advanced Care Planning, NHS, UK

1. AIMS[5]

"The area of advance care planning is becoming increasingly important but can be confusing for health and social care professionals and the public. ACP has always been an intrinsic part of the NHS End-of-life Care Programme (EoLC); the Preferred Priorities for Care (PPC) document is an example of this. Interest is growing, with more literature being published. The enactment of the Mental Capacity Act 2005 has highlighted the need for clarification and a national approach. The first edition of the document was initially developed as part of the three year (2004-2007) End-of-life Care Programme hosted by the NHS. Following feedback and debate the National End-of-life Care steering group met during 2006 and agreed that guidance relating to ACP was required for health and social care professionals which recognises their different contributions to an individual's care. We were grateful for the opportunity to consult and discuss with key stakeholders and a wider reference group and address three objectives:

1. To clarify the definition of ACP and related terms
2. To provide practical guidance on core competences, education and training of different professional groups and related ethical and legal implications

---

[5] The following is an adaption of Advance Care Planning by NHS UK. http://www.ncpc.org.uk/sites/default/files/AdvanceCarePlanning.pdf

3. To suggest next steps, to report on related work and suggest further work"

Difference between various terminology

Advance care planning

ACP is a process of discussion between an individual and their care providers irrespective of discipline. The difference between ACP and planning more generally is that the process of ACP is to make clear a person's wishes and will usually take place in the context of an anticipated deterioration in the individual's condition in the future, with attendant loss of capacity to make decisions and/or ability to communicate wishes to others.

With the individual's agreement, discussions should be:

- documented
- regularly reviewed
- communicated to key persons involved in their care
- If the individual wishes, their family and friends may be included.

Examples of what an ACP discussion might include are:

- the individual's concerns
- their important values or personal goals for care
- their understanding about their illness and prognosis, as well as particular preferences for types of care or treatment that may be beneficial in the future and the availability of these.

Statement of wishes and preferences

This is a summary term embracing a range of written and/or recorded oral expressions, by which people can, if they wish, write down or tell people about their wishes or preferences in relation to future treatment and care, or explain their feelings, beliefs and values that govern how they make decisions. They may cover medical and non-medical matters. They are not legally binding but should be used when determining a person's best interests in the event they lose capacity to make those decisions.

Advance decision
An advance decision must relate to a refusal of specific medical treatment and can specify circumstances. It will come into effect when the individual has lost capacity to give or refuse consent to treatment.

Careful assessment of the validity and applicability of an advance decision is essential before it is used in clinical practice. Valid advance decisions, which are refusals of treatment, are legally binding. Lasting Power of Attorney A Lasting Power of Attorney (LPA) is a statutory form of power of attorney created by the MCA (2005). Anyone who has the capacity to do so may choose a person (an 'attorney') to take decisions on their behalf if they subsequently lose capacity

2. Advance Care Planning
2.1. *Definition* Advance Care Planning (ACP) is a voluntary process of discussion about future care between an individual and their care providers, irrespective of discipline. If the individual wishes, their family and friends may be included. It is recommended that with the individual's agreement this discussion is documented, regularly reviewed, and communicated to key persons involved in their care[6]. An ACP discussion might include:

- the individual's concerns and wishes,
- their important values or personal goals for care,
- their understanding about their illness and prognosis,
- their preferences and wishes for types of care or treatment that may be beneficial in the future and the availability of these.

2.2. *Role of ACP in supportive care* If an individual wishes, ACP may be an integral part of the care and communication process and of their regular care plan review. The difference between ACP and care planning more generally is that the process of ACP will usually take place in the context of an anticipated deterioration in the individual's condition in the future, with attendant loss of capacity to make decisions and/or ability to communicate wishes to others.

2.3. *Documentation of ACP* There is no set format for making a record of advance care planning discussions, although having a person's wishes documented will prove helpful to those involved in their future

[6] See also NICE guidelines 2004 on Supportive and Palliative Care

care. Professionals who support a person in advance care planning should try to avoid following a rigid prescriptive method of interview and recording of discussions, this can be achieved by using an open question style of dialogue.

2.4. *ACP and the MCA* For individuals with capacity it is their current wishes about their care which needs to be considered. Under the MCA of 2005, individuals can continue to anticipate future decision-making about their care or treatment should they lack capacity. In this context, the outcome of ACP may be the completion of a statement of wishes and preferences or if referring to refusal of specific treatment may lead onto an advance decision to refuse treatment (Chapter 9, MCA 2005, Code of Practice).

This is not mandatory or automatic and will depend on the person's wishes. Alternatively, an individual may decide to appoint a person to represent them by choosing a person (an 'attorney') to take decisions on their behalf if they subsequently lose capacity (Chapter 5, MCA 2005, Code of Practice). A statement of wishes and preferences is not legally binding. However, it does have legal standing and must be taken into account when making a judgement in a person's best interests. Careful account needs to be taken of the relevance of statements of wishes and preferences when making best interest decisions (Chapter 5, MCA 2005, Code of Practice).

If an advance decision to refuse treatment has been made it is a legally binding document if that advance decision can be shown to be valid and applicable to the current circumstances. If it relates to life sustaining treatment it must be a written document which is signed and witnessed.

In all cases, an individual's contemporaneous capacity must be assessed on a decision-by decision basis. An individual may retain the ability to make a simple decision but not more complex decisions (Chapter 4, MCA 2005, Code of Practice).

2.5. *Considering the use of ACP: timing and context* ACP may be instigated by either the individual or a care provider at any time not necessarily in the context of illness progression but may be at one of the following key points in the individual's life:

- Life changing event, e.g. the death of spouse or close friend or relative
- Following a new diagnosis of life limiting condition eg cancer or motor neurone disease

- Significant shift in treatment focus e.g. chronic renal failure where options for treatment require review
- Assessment of the individual's needs
- Multiple hospital admissions
- Initiation of ACP discussion by a care provider requires careful consideration:
- ACP is voluntary and should not be initiated simply as part of routine record keeping or care
- The care provider may respond to 'cues' which indicate a desire to make specific wishes known e.g. worries about who will care for them
- ACP should not be initiated as a result of outside pressure e.g. family wishes or organisational pressures
- The care provider will require appropriate communication skills
- The care provider should have full knowledge of the person's medical condition, treatment options and social situation
- There may be someone more appropriate to carry out this discussion e.g. specialist nurse
- The time and setting should be appropriate for a private discussion

The pathway overseas is the one used in the NHS and the pathways recognised in this document.

NHS End-of-life Care Pathway
Note that there is no definitions of end-of-life; however, research supports either the presence of a chronic disease(s) or symptoms or functional impairments that persist but may also fluctuate, or, that the symptoms or impairments resulting from the underlying irreversible disease that require formal either paid professional or informal unpaid or volunteer care and can lead to death.

3. Statement of wishes, preferences, and values
Sometimes people will want to write down or tell others their wishes and preferences for future treatment and care, or explain their feelings or values that govern how they make decisions. Statements of wishes and preferences or documented conversations the person has had with

Pathway towards advanced care planning

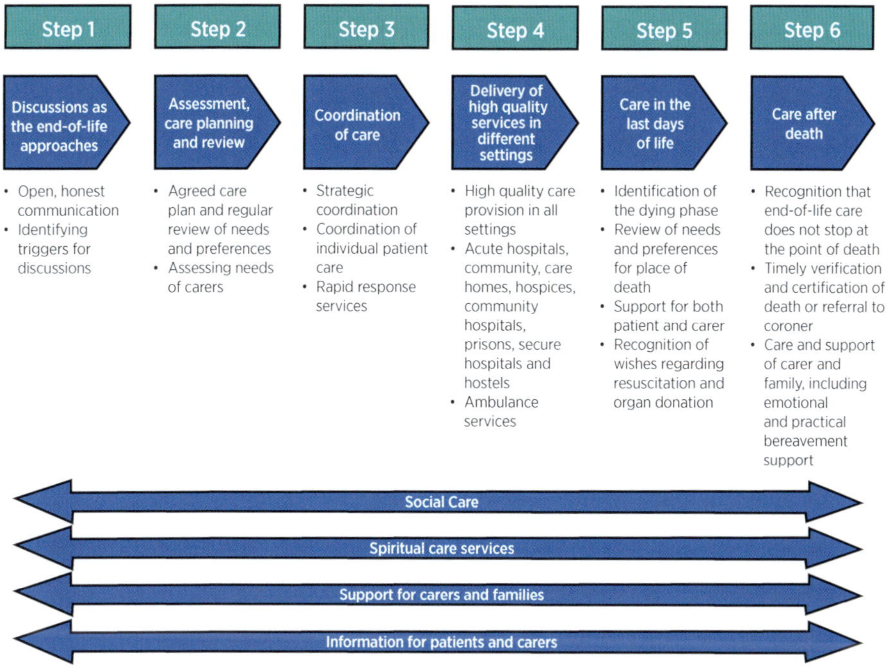

their family or other carers may be recorded in the person's notes. A statement of wishes and preferences can be of various types, for example:

- A requesting statement reflecting an individual's aspirations and preferences. This can help health and social care professionals identify how the person would like to be treated without binding them to that course of action if it conflicts with professional judgement (see section 3.1 ACP)
- A statement of the general beliefs and aspects of life which an individual values. This might provide a biographical portrait of the individual that subsequently aids deciding his/her best interests. Statements of wishes and preferences can include personal preferences, such as where one would wish to live, having a shower rather than a bath, or wanting to sleep with the light on. Sometimes people may wish to express their values e.g. that the welfare of their spouse or children is taken into account when decisions are made about their place of care. Sometimes people may have views about treatments they do not wish to receive but do not want to formalise these views as a specific advance decision to refuse treatment. These views should be

considered when acting in a person's best interests but will not be legally binding. A statement of wishes and preferences cannot be made in relation to any act which is illegal e.g. assisted suicide.

3.1. *Professional responsibilities in relation to statements of wishes and preferences* Under the MCA, anybody making a decision about the care or treatment of an individual, who has been assessed as lacking the capacity to make that decision for himself, will be required to take any statement of wishes and preferences into account when assessing that person's best interests. Part of assessing best interests should include making reasonable efforts to find out what a person's wishes, preferences, values and beliefs might be. This is likely to involve contacting the person's family or other care providers. They may be able to advise whether any statements of wishes or preferences exists or for help in determining that person's wishes. This will not always be possible, e.g. if an individual is admitted as an emergency, is unconscious and requires rapid treatment.

3.2 *Acting in a person's 'best interests'* A person assessing an individual's best interests must:

- Not make any judgement using the professional's view of the individual's quality of life
- Consider all relevant circumstances and options without discrimination
- Not be motivated by a desire to bring about an individual's death
- Consult with family partner or representative as to whether the individual previously had expressed any opinions or wishes about their future care e.g. ACP
- Consult with the clinical team caring for the individual
- Consider any beliefs or values likely to influence the individual if they had capacity
- Consider any other factors the individual would consider if they were able to do so
- Consider the individual's feelings

4. Teamwork and multidisciplinarity at the end-of-life

Evidence suggests a number of features that contribute to effective multidisciplinary working in end-of-life care:[7]

[7] National end-of-life programme 2012, UK.

- Ensuring wide representation at the multidisciplinary team meeting
- Each service/organisation having the capacity to respond rapidly and appropriately to changes in an individual's circumstances
- Streamlined discharge planning from hospital to home with fast tracking of continuing care and support at home
- Good communication systems to keep all members of the multidisciplinary team across all sectors fully informed, including community, health and social care services
- Knowing whom to contact in each relevant organisation
- Having a structure in place for someone's advance care plan to be updated and communicated
- Having procedures in place to support ethical decision-making and reaching informed consent

NICE guidelines on end-of-life care

1. People approaching the end-of-life are identified in a timely way.
2. People approaching the end-of-life and their families and carers are communicated with, and offered information, in an accessible and sensate way in response to their needs and preferences.
3. People approaching the end-of-life are offered comprehensive holistic assessments in response to their changing needs and preferences, with the opportunity to discuss, develop and review a personalized care plan for current and future support and treatment.
4. People approaching the end-of-life have their physical and specific psychological needs safely, effectively and appropriately met at any time of day or nights, including access to medicine and equipment.
5. People approaching the end-of-life are offered timely personalised support for their social, practical and emotional needs, which is appropriate to their preferences and maximises independence and social participation for as long as possible.
6. People approaching the end-of-life are offered spiritual and religious support appropriate to their needs and preferences.
7. Families and carers of people approaching the end-of-life are offered comprehensive holistic assessments in response

to their changing needs and preferences, and holistic support appropriate to their current needs and preferences.

8. People approaching the end-of-life receive consistent care that is coordinated effectivel across all relevant settings and services at any time of day of night, and delivered by practitioners who are aware of the person's current medical condition, care plan, and preferences.
9. People approaching the end-of-life who experience a crisis at any time of day or night receive prompt, safe and effective urgent care appropriate to their needs and preferences.
10. People approaching the end-of-life who may benefit from specialist palliative care are offered this care in a timely way appropriate to their needs and preferences, at any time of day or night.
11. People in the last days of life are identified in a timely way and have their care coordinated and delivered in accordance with their personalised care plan, including rapid access to holistic support, equipment and administration of medication.
12. The body of a person who has died is cared for in a culturally sensitive and dignified manner.
13. Families and carers of people who have died receive timely verification and certification of death.
14. People closely affected by a death are communicated with in a sensitive way and are offered immediate and ongoing bereavement, emotional and spiritual support appropriate to their needs and preferences.
15. Health and social care workers have the knowledge, skills and attitudes necessary to be competent to provide high quality care and support for people approaching the end-of-life and their families and carers.
16. Generalists and specialist services providing care for people approaching the end-of-life and their families and carers have a multidisciplinary workforce sufficient in number and skill mix to provide high-quality care and support.

It should be noted that the above in no way introduces the legal concept of an Advance Directive, but yet supports the whole concept of a Advanced Care Planning. The two titles ought not to be confused because of the common word 'advance/advanced'.

Assessing need and coordination of care[8]

1. Every care plan should be based on an assessment of need. In the absence of individual needs assessment, a meaningful care plan incorporating support tailored to the individual is not possible.
2. The person's preferences regarding both the type of care they would wish to receive and the setting or location in which they wish to be cared for should be elicited.
3. The care plan should be recorded with input from the multidisciplinary team. This ensures that both the assessment and care plan are comprehensive and identify ways in which the needs can be addressed.
4. Services must be coordinated around the care plan for the individual, as without a coordinated joined-up approach there is a risk that the needs will not be met well or that people could fall through a gap in service provision.
5. There should be regular review of the person's needs and preferences and their care plan, as their deteriorating condition may lead to changes in both needs and choices.
6. People should have rapid access to re-assessment and care as their neds change, including access to equipment or additional care support to ensure that people do not revolve back unnecessarily to hospitals or health care provision.
7. A financial assessment should be included within the assessment, particularly in relation to benefits and entitlements.

Principles of the consensus statement of the Erasmus+ project, EndCare, University of Malta

1. One must give patients approaching the end-of-life the same quality of care as all other patients. Patients must be treated with dignity, respect and compassion, as must those close to them, especially when facing difficult questions about decision-making in the care of the dying person. Privacy and rights to confidentiality must be respected and also the right to spiritual care.

[8] See Chapter 3, "Assessing Need and Planning Care", *Pathways through care at the end-of-life*, Hayes, A., et al.

2. There must be no discrimination based on the patient being older, having a disability or those who understandably may be referred to as 'social cases'. It is recognised that internationally as well as perhaps locally, some of these groups have experienced inequality in getting access to health services.
3. Health professionals caring for dying people must be aware of the main provisions on basic rights and principles expressed in the Convention on Human Rights and Biomedicine of the Council of Europe which provides also for the expression in advance of wishes of patients concerning the end of their lives, as long as these are within the remits of local law.
4. Hospital structures for documenting any wishes which plan ahead (Advanced Care Planning) ought to be put in place for the efficient and effective communication between health professionals.
5. There is a presumption in favour of prolonging life following established ethical and legal principles. However there is no absolute obligation to prolong life irrespective of the consequences to the patient and irrespective of the patient's views.
6. It is important to keep in mind that:
    - One cannot treat without the patient's consent and that patients have a right to refuse treatment, including life-prolonging treatment
    - There is a difference between killing and allowing someone to die when death is the inevitable outcome
    - One need not give disproportionate or futile treatment, or treatment which is considered extraordinary, especially by the patient.
    - One can give appropriate pain relief and if necessary even sedation, even if these shorten life.
    - It is the patient who decides what is considered as 'ordinary' or 'extraordinary' treatment or care for himself or herself.
7. One must assume that every adult patient has the capacity (as defined in the Mental Health Act of the Laws of Malta) (DATE) to make decisions about their care and treatment. If a patient's capacity is limited, one must provide all the necessary support and help to maximise their ability to understand and weigh information. When capacity is impaired the one must see who is making decision

on the patient's behalf. Decisions doctors and relatives make must ensure the overall benefit of the patient, including options not to treat. Doctors must consult close with relatives, especially where wishes by the patient have been expressed or even documented.

8. People or relatives may therefore be afraid that high doses of pain relief which may shorten life are active euthanasia, or, that removing a treatment which is extraordinary, disproportionate or even futile, is a form of passive euthanasia. In this case there is the necessity to explain that there is no conflict of values as one is not deliberately bringing about, directly or indirectly, the death of the patient.
9. One should aim to reach a consensus through mediation and if necessary ask patients and relatives to consider speaking with a learned member or representative of their faith.
10. It is important to note that monotheistic religions, including Christian, Muslim and Judaic all agree on the above principles.
11. Families may conversely request measures which go beyond normal medical wisdom, or even make requests which are unreasonable, such as keeping someone on a life support system when there is not hope for improvement or when there is already a diagnosis of brain death.
12. It is important to realise that although removing treatment and support systems is emotionally more difficult (for relatives and health professionals alike) than deciding not to start treatment or measure in the first instance, a principle of moral equivalence exists, that is, they are legally and morally equivalent.
13. Clear communication is the key to effective conflict resolution and legal advice should be a last option.
14. Mediation is the most important and efficient route to resolving conflict, especially where there are differences in the cultures of patients, families, and health providers. Mediation may have to involve an ethicist who will:
    - Identify the parties to the conflict
    - Understand the stated and latent interests of the parties
    - Level the playing field to minimise disparities of power, knowledge, skill, and experience
    - Search for common ground, especially one that is time-sensitive
    - Ensure that the consensus reached is a 'principled resolution' in light of legal rights and ethical scholarship

- Follow up to be sure that the agreement reached has sufficient structural supports to become the reality of care (Neveroff Dubler, 2005).

15. The promotion of these principles are to be encouraged by politicians, patient groups and social groups and institutions (including religious, associations and patient NGOs) and adequate knowledge and training should be provided where necessary.

Royal College of Physicians, UK,
Advance Care Planning table:

Guideline Development Process Advance Table Care Planning

These guidelines have been developed in accordance with the principles laid down by the AGREE collaboration (Appraisal of Guidelines for Research and Evaluation).

Scope and purpose

The scope	
Overall objectives of the guidelines	The objective of the Guideline Development Group was to inform health and social care professionals on how best to manage ACP in clinical practice.
The patient group covered	The guidelines focus on adults, with particular emphasis on older people. Relevant evidence from all countries will be considered, but the guidelines will reflect the legal situation in England and Wales. ADRTs relating to psychiatric treatment would be excluded, as would any papers concerning minors (<18 years old).
Target audience	All clinicians, including general physicians, GPs and other health and social care professionals

Clinical areas/questions covered

Attitudes

1. Is the general public in favour of ACP?
2. What are the attitudes of health care professionals towards ACP?

Barriers

3. How often do individuals change their minds about ACP?
4. Does ACP increase mortality?
5. Does ACP deny access to appropriate health care?
6. How can uptake of ACP be improved?

Communication

7. When should ACP discussion take place?
8. Where should ACP discussion take place?
9. What are the best methods for communicating about ACPs with individuals?
10. What is the optimal method for communicating about ACP within families?
11. What are the optimal methods for ensuring that ACPs are available at the point of care, especially in emergency settings?
12. What are the optimal methods to ensure ACP documents are noted in health care records and are available to healthcare practitioners seeing the patient for the first time?

Content

13. Should people preparing ACP documents use values statements or be more specific in their guidance?
14. Do patients change their healthcare decision in a given situation?
15. How often should advance care planning decisions/statements be reviewed?
16. How recent does an ACP document need to be in order to remain valid?

Demand

17. How many individuals have completed advance care plans in England and Wales? How does this compare internationally?
18. Who is using ACP?
19. Who does not use ACP and why not?

Health care proxies

20. Do LPAs influence care?
21. What is the concordance between surrogates and patients?
22. How accurate are substitute judgements in ACP?

Outcomes

23. Can ACP improve health care choice concordance?
24. Does ACP affect satisfaction with health care?
25. Can ACP improve the quality of end-of-life care?
26. What are the costs of an ACP programme?
27. What additional benefits do ACP discussions offer apart from directing care?

Role of health care professionals

28. Which health care professionals should be involved in ACP?

Training

29. What are the training needs of health care professionals, including care home sector staff?
30. What are the optimal methods for delivering ACP training and awareness to health care professionals?

Dementia

31. What is known about ACP in people with dementia?

Downloads

Concise Guidance to Good Practice: file:///C:/Users/User/Downloads/Concise%20advance%20care%20planning%20guidelines%20(2).pdf

Stakeholder involvement

The Guideline Development Group (GDG)	The guideline committee was made up of various stakeholders, including strong lay representation, general practice and other clinicians. Organisations represented on guideline committee included the British Geriatrics Society, the Faculty of Old Age Psychiatry, Royal College of Psychiatrists, the Royal College of General Practitioners, the National Council for Palliative Care and the Royal College of Nursing. Additional input was given by palliative care physicians. Users were represented through the involvement of Alzheimer's Society, Age Concern, Help the Aged and the patient representative panel of the Royal College of Physicians.
Funding	These guidelines were commissioned by the Clinical Practice and Evaluation Committee of the British Geriatrics Society. Funding was obtained from the British Geriatrics Society.
Conflicts of Interest	No external funding has been sought or obtained. All authors and group members have declared that they have no actual or potential conflicts of interest

Rigour of development

Evidence gathering	The following databases were searched: OVID MEDLINE(R) (1966+), EMBASE (1980+), PsychINFO (1967+), BNI (1985+), HMIC (July 2006), CINAHL (1982+), AMED (1985+) The systematic review consisted of two phases. The first phase (scoping exercise) identified evidence from sources least susceptible to bias. A comprehensive search strategy was used to identify all eligible randomised controlled trials, previous systematic reviews, and existing evidence-based guidelines. The second phase searched for evidence from studies more prone to bias (cohort studies, case-control studies and where relevant, surveys). Where evidence was lacking for a specific question, additional sources were examined including case reports, literature reviews, and evidence from expert opinion or consensus. Special attention was given to non-research publications, such as government reports, including the Mental Capacity Act and the accompanying Code of Practice. Scoping exercise Grading of evidence during the scoping exercise followed the principles used by the Scottish Intercollegiate Guideline Network [SIGN] and the National Institute of Clinical Excellence [NICE]. The reviewers felt that the SIGN appraisal tool did not lend itself well to the papers being examined, and following external consultation the guideline development committee agreed to change to using the appraisal tool developed for use in the NSF for Long Term Conditions.[140]

Links between evidence and recommendations	A set of key questions to help guide the literature search were identified by the guideline development group and these were incorporated into the search criteria along with the generic search terms. Evidence based summary statements were derived from the literature and used to develop the guidelines at a series of consensus meetings.
Piloting and peer review	The Clinical Effectiveness and Evaluation Unit of the Royal College of Physicians reviewed the methodology and reviewed the final guidance prior to publication. All stakeholder organisations were asked to ratify and co-badge the final guidelines. Formal external reviews were obtained from Professor Jane Seymour (Nottingham), Professor Peter Bartlett (Nottingham) and Professor Gideon Caplan (New South Wales, Australia).

Chapter 11
Comparing Islam and Christian end-of-life moral guidelines[1]

This paper tends to identify common ground between the Islamic and Christian cultures. Since these two cultures are more and more coming to live in the same countries, it is important to acknowledge common ground since the laws of countries apply to all. The paper will go through several issues, including the stopping of futile treatment, the administration of ordinary and extraordinary care, defining the difference between death and allowing one to die, and indeed accepting death as sometimes being an inevitable and acceptable outcome. The paper will also discuss palliative care including pain relief and sedation. From here one delves into the case of Persistent Vegetative States and the morality of over-enthusiastic treatment which pushes people into this state.

One will focus on the differences, such as passive euthanasia and analyze whether this is merely a difference of interpreting terms. There is also a phenomenon in some countries querying the removal futile treatment and perhaps lack of a legal framework. At least one study shows concern with religious moral grounds. In conclusion one attempts to identify the common grounds on the end-of-life and whether indeed morality and laws in this regard is guided by religious positions. It is perhaps important that laws respect the moral normative values of populations, especially with pressure coming for more liberal positions. Even if the latter are introduced in many countries, such as euthanasia, the discussion of which is not the scope of this paper, it is important that health care (and legislation) recognizes the more

[1] Mallia, P., "A practical comparison between Islamic and Christian end-of-life moral guidelines towards harmonisation of end-of-life care", in Aquilina, K., Mallia, P., Ellul, B. (eds.) *Contemporary issues in Maltese Medical Ethics and Law*, University of Malta Press, Malta, 2017, pp. 112-132.

common moral ground, the lack of which may be leading to more suffering.

Introduction

With the internationalization and globalization of medicine and its advancement in being able to keep people on life support end-of-life necessitated strong reviews. The concept of whether one should keep someone on life support until brain death was challenged early on in the case of Karen Ann Quinlan – a case which is recognized as a historical landmark finding its citation in the Routledge Encyclopedia of the History of Medicine (Bynum & Porter, 2001) and which was the first case in which an American court of law recognized the teaching of a traditional religion over and above scientific learning (in this case waiting until Karen would have been brain-dead).

By 'internationalization' one refers to the transfer of people between countries. Immigrant doctors, or those who become doctors, will generally inherit traditional customs and religions which are thus imported into countries which become multicultural. This is a phenomenon, for example (but not limited to), of ex-colonial countries, for example, who travel to the United Kingdom and still have 'Royal College' membership examination. Many others go to the United States. End-of-life decisions are carried into cultures and different Christian and Muslim countries have had to evaluate these decisions according to their culture and religious perspectives and reach conclusions. Although there are subtle differences and at time disagreements, on the whole one sees that there is a general agreement, but as seen here, different definitions, most notably when it comes to defining passive euthanasia can create confusion.

Conversely, with the increasing scope of globalization (which is the spread of cultures across geographical areas and which includes the increase in communication and more easily available and faster means of movement of people), a harmonization of end-of-life morality is also deemed necessary in order to arrive at coherent 'clinical ethics' judgements giving us a more 'global ethcs'. It is not merely the religious and philosophical questions that should concern us however, but the actual practice and when and where it fails and why. However the scope of this paper is the former; the latter has been accepted as an Erasmus+ proposal which is to commence in the fall of 2015 (Mallia, 2015). Before harmonization is accepted one has to recon with the challenge of cultures and religious points of view and whether indeed there is any form of agreement on the main issues. For example Walker and Lovat (2015) have made a point of proposing the concept of ordinary versus extraordinary treatment as being an ideal path in most situations, including cultural. Conflict is not however that easy to resolve as it often arises because of difference in values; it is not merely a dispute. You can resolve a number of disputes with the main conflict remaining there (Tillett, 2002). It is perhaps the lack of understanding of the underlying values which people hold, including health care professionals, which may be of the main concern. Does my religion allow me to terminate this treatment or to remove this drug which the doctor is saying is futile?

In arriving at some form of resolution a comparative analysis between the various cultural/religious points of view is important. One appreciates that religions have been on the avant-garde of these moral issues. Here the aim is to deliberately compare the Christian and Muslim religions, appreciating that the Judeo-Christian model would have served as well. Of course one admits that other religions play an important role but these two major religions, which have often found themselves at loggerheads on theological points, find themselves interacting more and more. There is probably more positive interactions than the media or extremist groups would want the world to believe and it is interesting to observe the overlap. Truth telling, although a compelling cultural issue is not discussed in this paper as it focuses more on religious moral teaching; pain relief, futile treatment and extraordinary treatment.

Method

The methodology used was not to compare various theological positions from both religions. Given that theologians can provide interesting perspectives in both camps, these are ongoing dialogues and do not reflect official (or traditional) positions which can, at the end of the day, help clinicians, patients and their families understand what can and cannot be done on moral grounds at the end-of-life without breaching their cultural and religious values. This is important from a clinical ethics perspective and therefore the main methodology used here is a search for authors who have discussed the more official positions of the respective positions. The literature and sources which discuss the official positions was therefore consulted. It is important to note that a small separation has been made under Christian denominations – namely the Catholic and other Christian denominations at points. The reason is that when referring to Christianity we refer to a cluster of different denominations (including Catholic), some of which tend to be post-traditional (Engelhardt & Smith Iltis, 2005). As done in a review on and of life by *The Lancet* in 2005 in which the Catholic point of view was treated separately, it was felt that reference to Catholic traditions sometimes merited to be distinguished from the general group of 'Christian'. This should be understood further in the next paragraph.

Respective backgrounds on life

Many papers which have analyzed end-of-life issues from the Islamic Perspective invariably and rightly-so start from the underlying religious concept of life and death. (Sachedina, 2005; Bagheri, 2013; & AtiGhetchi, 2007).

Muslims believe they were created to discover God's work in the universe and to appreciate and serve God's ends. From time to time God sends prophets, and the prophet Mohammed, founder of Islam, is the last one in this line of prophets. Life belongs to God and its willful termination is therefore prohibited. Neither however must one not accept death. Practices of euthanasia, voluntary or involuntary, are thus prohibited. The debatable questions arose mostly in the context of health care, especially with hospitalized patients who may or may not be given care which can be considered extraordinary. Muslim legal scholars are under pressure to respond to questions relating to health care with the onset of advancing medical technology (*ibid.*). This is especially so in questions relating to end-of-life. Their deliberations fall under the auspices of the Islamic Juridical Council (IJC) which is an organ of the Organisation of Islamic Conference (OIC), in which jurists from different schools of thought respond coherently to specific problems and situations. These are published in a quarterly journal issued by the IJC. The Quran recognizes the limits of human nature, and that pain is a form of test or trial. We shall see that this has not prevented the use of pain relief; however, also because jurists agree that traditional Islamic teaching cannot cater for new circumstances and developments. Islam is inherently discursive and pluralistic (*ibid.*).

One finds the same debates in Islam that one finds among Christians on end-of-life. However the latter is complicated by the ambiguity of the term Christian, which encompasses a number of groups which 'at best' share resemblances (Engelhardt & Smith Iltis, 2005). There are Unitarians, Seventh-ay Adventists, Anglicans, Mormons, Lutherans, Orthodox, etc., not to mention Catholic. These groups differ in theology and indeed on end-of-life decisions. However, many Christian groups can also be seen as traditional, and whilst these will, for example, not accept euthanasia, the post-traditional groups, such as the Unitarian, will accept it. According to Engelhardt, a failure to acknowledge difference amongst Christians can lead to end-of-life decisions which patients and families will reject. Christianity has always affirmed the importance of health care but since the constructions of the first hospitals, there has always been intense discourse on new developments. Miller, in his book on 'The Birth of the Hospital in the Byzantine Empire' (Miller, 1997) points out that although Christianity became a pioneer in the cure of the sick in hospitals, and religious orders were dedicated to being 'hospitallers' bringing the practice of medicine in a 'thoroughly Christian environment'. There were however many Christians who at the time of the first hospitals felt that pagan science was entering Christianity and that the only healer was Christ himself. This was especially so for the Byzantine Christians. Eventually Alexandrian theologians of the third century and the Greek Fathers of the fourth gave their blessing to medicine, giving it a paragon of charity.

Today's Catholic religion also finds different theological and philosophical methodologies resulting in differences of opinion; but one tends to find coherence on end-of-life issues (Markwell, 2005). Catholics are thought to remain attuned to the message of Christ and pain is also seen as being redemptory. This also gave rise to the controversy on sedation at the end-of-life, which may inhibit a dying patient from making redemptive attempts. Markwell points out that two basic values predominate in Catholics bioethics – that of human dignity, and the interconnectedness of every individual. The human person is called into a relationship with God. Theologians have discussed end-of-life issues at least since the 16th century where extraordinary measures meant also that families needed not to go through expense which they could hardly afford to cure the ill. This is discussed further below. However Catholics see that bodily life is not an absolute good to be preserved at all costs and that God participates in the human condition through Jesus Christ who is His incarnation. The value of charity and solidarity demands, however, that one responds to the needs of others, especially the poor and needy, including the sick. This is why the doctor-patient relationship is seen better as a covenant rather than a contract and is the reason for virtue ethics being given prominence over principlism more recently (Pellegrino, 2009).

Christians (in general) prohibit all forms of assisted suicide and forbid saving life at all costs. Catholicism believes in the sanctity of life, as a gift and creation of God. One does not own one's body. We have seen that amongst protestant groups some have advocated for passive euthanasia. We shall see that whilst there may be general agreement of active euthanasia there is a problem with passive euthanasia as seen in the Islamic tradition; although one accepts removal of futile treatment as important in general it still falls under a category of passive euthanasia which is granted an exception 49 in (Zahedi, Larijani & Tavakoly Bazzaz, 2007). This merits some analysis in the paragraph on extraordinary care when trying to reconcile teaching to form common moral ground globally in order not to be caught in definitions.

It is also noteworthy that the Catholic Church gave its teaching a more formal form in 1952 when Pope Pius XII made a clear and ample clarification to doctors. This was important for Western countries which were predominantly Catholic. But this does not mean that Catholics do not differ nowadays – mostly it is a matter of either ignorance of what the Church has actually been saying and indeed a difference in interpreting the teaching. The case of Karen Ann Quinlan was indeed a historical case because it was the first time in the United States that the court upheld a religious (Catholoc) teaching of extraordinary care (as that of a social institution) as opposed to the scientific 'teaching' that death on life support is seen through the concept of 'brain death', following a series of tests to ascertain this. Thus Quinlan was not scientifically dead but was admitted to being given extraordinary treatment which was keeping her alive in a futile sense. One wonders whether this would have been possible without the 1952 assertion. Even giving too much treatment and pushing patients into a vegetative state was seen as morally wrong and repudiated under Pope Paul VI (Petrini, 2011).

But paradoxically the more recent controversy over artificial nutrition and hydration (ANH) has brought about the concept that unless physiologically futile or burdensome, people in PVS should be given ANH (Shannon & Kockler, 2009, p. 153), even though (therefore) there was a window of opportunity, as it were, when the patient was at a stage in which he/she could have been taken off life support - keeping in mind of course that persistent vegetative states are always a side effect of over enthusiastic medical care.

Catholic doctrine however is clear on the main concepts but interpreting the Magisterium, which is the formal teaching of the Catholic Church (Magisterium of the Catholic Church, 1994) has proved problematic with Artificial Nutrition and Hydration (ANH), what is futile, and how much one ought to treat people who are in danger of falling into a Persistent Vegetative State (PVS) or are already diagnosed in such a condition. Whilst therefore in 1952 it was asserted that one cannot treat patients without their formal consent or without the consent of the family if the patient is unable to make decisions, and that it is the patient who decides what ought to be extraordinary or not for him, more recent declarations have sought to make hydration as an 'ordinary' care. Although there have been clarifications by the Church, many practices in hospitals fear removing a hydration with most people dying with a drip still attached to their arms, not taking into consideration the discomfort it may produce inherently or simply to insert another needle in order to maintain it (Ballatt & Campling, 2013).

Paternalism vs rights

To emphasis the misconceptions on how people interpret morality and perhaps the predominant paternalism in maintaining some treatment whilst withholding other, one need only look again at PVS. It is interesting that whilst ANH is advocated in PVS, many then assume that giving an antibiotic may be extraordinary and not necessary. This is paradoxical and perhaps immoral. It really depends on the policy of the hospital on how to deal with PVS and the budget one has for doing so. If one is keeping a PVS patient alive because of human dignity why should not one treat the flu or an infection? Clearly the 'fight' against death has given rise to PVS being almost accepted and no one seems to question the moral implication (or whether it is indeed morally wrong) to over-treat a patient to the point of sending him or her into a vegetative state. Conversely, Robert Veatch has indeed pointed out that when relatives of dying patients challenge medics and hospitals who wish to remove futile treatment, courts in the United States have been willing to accede to the wishes of the relatives (Veatch, 2013). He notes that in the 70's, families fought for the right to refuse medical treatments which were seen merely as prolonging the dying process. The situation has changed over the years with families challenging doctors who believe that the treatment is futile. There is a paradigm shift therefore from physiological futility to normative futility – a futility which is discussed on a rights and philosophical basis rather than an epistemological and physiological basis. It should be pointed out however that this article avoids this argument, which may perhaps, it is contended, arise due to lack of moral education on the part of the public (i.e. a lack of understanding what their own religion is saying, presuming that adhere to one). From a liberal perspective there is little one can do but to appeal to a more secular ethic, arguing and explaining futility as was done in the 70's – that it merely prolongs the agony.

One will now critically appraise specific aspects of end-of-life care in order to tease out the common moral ground in the hope of a harmonization which may help multicultural societies and on broader grounds, harmonization.

Killing and allowing to die

Both Christian and Islamic traditions distinguish between killing and allowing to die. AtiGhetchi explains that every Muslim doctor must take all effort to save a patient from dying *if the probabilities of success* appear significant and that on the contrary artificially prolonging the vegetative state of a person is unlawful as it is consciousness that makes an individual responsible (AtiGhetchi, 2007, p. 271). This contrasts with Catholic teaching as stated above, notwithstanding that the Church had pronounced itself against pushing people into a vegetative state. Of course the perception that hospitalized care has become less and less 'extraordinary' may have an influence on this. The public perception of intensive care may indeed be accepted and demanded by relatives who do not have to pay for it directly.

Sachedina points out that the medical judgements about death are based on probability and a doctor can only predict that death is imminent when it is very close. He states that, 'Hence, the Qur'an offers a sober reminder that there are times when human beings need to recognize their own limits and entrust nature to take its own course (Qur'an 39:42)' (Sachedina, 2005, p. 776). Refusing to recognize that inevitability and naturalness of deaths leads to more aggressive treatments (which in turn can lead to a vegetative state), but however to withhold a specific intervention at a crucial time which may be life-saving results in "deliberate avoidance of responsibility". Life support, he asserts, can be turned off when physicians are certain about the inevitability of death.

Christians have long asserted that a doctor is not breaking any moral rule if on recognition that death is inevitable one allows a person to die (Hinton, 1967). Of course, this does not imply that one should forego life-saving treatment. It only means that prolonging life for the sake of fighting death is not good moral practice. In this regard one should consider the difference perhaps of various practices when people choose to die at home. It is understood that one cannot offer the same end-of-life care at home than one can in hospital. Unless there are good community palliative care services, one cannot have even intravenous lines for hydration although pain relief can easily be provided intramuscularly. So, it is understood that hospitalization can prolong a dying person's life by a few days. This practice is accepted in most Christian and Islamic countries. However, people can often choose that someone dies in hospital not only because of the burden of having a relative die at home but because they may feel they are doing their best for their relative. Once at hospital the medical team may feel obliged that this perception is respected and therefore inevitably intravenous lines go up for hydration and nutrition. One finds it difficult to accept the moral equivalence of removing these drips as it seems to deceive the end of doing one's best, notwithstanding that thrombosed veins can mean that the dying person is punctured by a needle several times each time one wants to re-insert a new venflow when the other has become blocked.

From a Muslim perspective, home death, as AtiGhetchi conversely points out (*ibid.*, p. 271), whilst many people feel that if for the dying person his or her environment makes the process less burdensome, homes do not have the 'modern clinical equipment' and therefore this inclination to keep the person at home is not without its 'problematic consequences'. Whilst sending someone to hospital can relieve the burden from the family, there is also the question whether this constitutes a 'discard' and therefore in 'insidious form of passive euthanasia'. He also points out that in Tunis, in order to avoid scenes by relatives at hospital, doctors may suggest that the dying patient is taken home, finding solace in a decree which allows this transfer if the patient or relatives request it. It is a matter of what is in the best interests of the patient. One does however notice the tensions between what is considered appropriate or disproportionate does give rise to doubt about whether this is some form of passive euthanasia. More will be pointed out in this regard within the Muslim tradition, but we have encountered it also within other traditions when speaking about appropriate hydration and the discomfort it may produce in maintaining it.

It seems therefore that there is no real moral contention about dying at home in each religion. In fact, many do prefer to die at home and can forego treatment on the mere basis that they may deem hospitalization itself to be burdensome. The relatives do indeed come into play when the person approaches death and is unable to communicate well. Their decision whether to send the patient to die in hospital may be based on burden or otherwise. Sometimes they cannot respect the patient's wish to die at home for practical reasons. For example, in the practice of the author an 86-year-old gentleman who was semiconscious refused nappies and each time he need to pass urine or stool, his daughter, who lived alone with him, needed to call in her uncles to help her lift him from bed. The patient did on this occasion die before being sent to hospital. The problem would have been twofold - that the patient's wish could not have been acceded, and that there would have been the risk that the patient be subjected to investigations, drips and so on.

Disproportionate treatment vs passive euthanasia

The Catholic, position on this issue are very clear (as evidenced above) (Magisterium of the Catholic Church, 1994): "Discontinuing medical procedures that are burdensome, dangerous, extraordinary, or disproportionate to the expected outcome can be legitimate; it is the refusal of 'over-zealous' treatment. Here one does not will to cause death; one's inability to impede it is merely accepted. The decisions should be made by the patient if he is competent and able or, if not, by those legally entitled to act for the patient, whose reasonable will and legitimate interests must always be respected."

Amongst Christians end-of-life decisions are sometimes controversial. Engelhardt and Smith Iltis point out that whilst some protestant groups clearly oppose euthanasia and assisted suicide, others accept passive but refuse active euthanasia. Still others accept active euthanasia as a personal choice. There is also controversy about withholding ANH as many see it as an intention to cause death. Traditional Christians (see introduction for distinction) never intentionally cause death. Catholic teaching on withholding or withdrawing treatment has been around at least since the 16th century, as pointed out above. Patients can choose what is ordinary and what is extraordinary (which includes excessive expense, pain or other inconvenience), especially if it does not offer reasonable hope. Markwell points out that 'ordinary' was originally used to mean 'what is medically customary' and perhaps this is the main problem with nutrition and hydration and even other methods which many view as extraordinary but which many (including doctors) have come to see as 'customary'. This of course creates problems beyond the mere cultural and religious but is more of a sociological tendency promulgated by the high hopes people have in hospitals and medicine and which can explain Veatch's observation that courts of law tend to agree with patients and relatives when hospitals decide to forego some treatment considered futile.

Whilst many countries like the United Kingdom have clarified end-of-life issues on their General Medical Council guidelines, other countries are not very clear at all. The main issue often is with ANH. Why this is so and why not have also ventilation is mysterious. After all oxygen is as important to life as water and nutrition and whilst dying people do not normally drink or eat, they usually are still breathing.

Indeed, dying of suffocation is probably more 'painful'. Yet cases in which people have legitimately refused artificial ventilation even when conscious are surrounded by controversy (Archdiocese of Atlanta, 1990). This practice has also been recognized in the UK (Howard & Bogle, 2005), whilst that of Dianne Pretty had been refused because her case was not one of refusal of treatment, as was the case for Mrs B who was permitted to refuse artificial ventilation. Conversely, in Italy, the Church did not recognize the same appeal of Mr Piergiorgio Welby. On the other hand medically assisted nutrition and hydration should be seen as optional if they become excessively burdensome and cause physical discomfort (United States Conference of Catholic Bishops, 2009). Clearly the issues restrict themselves to end-of-life only and not quality of life, although there are contradictions between the McAffee and the Welby cases. Clearly however, disproportionate or extraordinary care, and even that which is ordinary care that become burdensome and thus can be considered disproportionate are allowed under Catholic and other religions' moral guidance. It is not a case of passive euthanasia, as the same actions in a quality-of-life issue are.

There is a clear *difference of nomenclature* when one compares Islamic cases of disproportionate and burdensome treatment. Whereas generally these are allowed, it is still labeled by many authors as 'passive euthanasia'. Zadehi et al. (2007) point out that whilst some Muslim scholars assume that Islamic law permits the withdrawal of disproportionate treatment on the basis of the consent of the family, and whilst, as pointed out above, the Muslims distinguish between killing and allowing to die, killing is seen as euthanasia and allowing to die as passive euthanasia.

This distinction is pointed out by other authors writing on generally accepted Muslim teaching. Sachedina (2005, p. 776) points out that the distinction between "killing (active euthanasia) and letting die (passive euthanasia)" often distinguishes between 'suicide and foregoing treatment or between homicide and natural death'. He says that there are two important instances that "could be interpreted as passive assistance...but that would not result in criminal charges". These are pain relief and removing a death delaying treatment following discussion with the patient and/or the family. This is because death is inevitable. We have seen that AtiGhetchi has implied that for some, allowing people to die at home can be interpreted as passive euthanasia because they are denied hospital care. But he shows that this is not always practical and patients and families do seem to have a choice here as well. Yet the word 'passive euthanasia' is used in a negative sense as well. He again recognizes that most Muslim scholars will allow this passive euthanasia in case of futile treatment – whilst relatives "frequently request extreme treatment in the hope of recovery of a dying patient" and that whilst some Muslim scholars believe that "every possible effort should be made for the survival of the patient", "others introduce the categories of unnecessary, ineffective or inappropriate measure when the patient is in the final throes".

There is clearly a lack of guidelines on extraordinary measures in many countries of both denominations. Doctors may fear lack of legislation when it comes to removal of futile treatment (Ballatt & Campling, 2013, p. 116). Bagheri notes that the concept of futility has caused problems not only how to define what is futile but when and how to apply it (Bagheri, 2013, p. 264). Withholding and withdrawing life support in Iran is controversial but whilst there is a general dominancy of physicians (which Bagheri refers to as a medical paternalism – and hence of societal significance), the general idea among physicians is that medical futility should be based on physiological futility. It is thus not a value judgement but an objective one. Many physicians also emphasize the role of the family. Abuhasna and Abdulkareem Al Obaidi (2013) also argue for the need of legislation in the United Arab Emirates and they advocate for a national policy 'based on physicians' attitudes and the perception of patients' to clarify futile treatment and end-of-life decisions. These authors argue that there is growing awareness of the importance for guidelines on end-of-life issues and in general there is agreement that families should be involved in the decision-making process. They say that although from an Islamic perspective that are no clear guidelines on end-of-life care for the Muslim patient, many scholars agree that withdrawal of life support and futile treatment is acceptable in cases where physicians agree that the patient has died (p. 251). When it comes to futile treatment critical care physicians have argue that it is important to bring the family of the terminally ill patient on board and have advocated for "optimal education of patients and their families", which often resolve these issue. Perhaps by optimal education they refer mostly to good communication and empathy. In general, they say that there is a growing understanding of medical futility in UAE countries.

As a final example of an Islamic country, Turkey presents an interesting position. There is no legislation which covers end-of-life removal of futile treatment (Arda & Aciduman, 2013). Discussions on DNR orders are usually between physicians themselves according to cited studies. A Medical Deontology Regulation of 1960 makes it very difficult for physicians to limit or withdraw life support (p. 242). In fact there is no law which covers medical futility and that allow the withdrawal of treatment considered to be futile. Whilst euthanasia is considered a crime it is not the case that on a daily practice, "it is possible to state that passive euthanasia is exercised in certain cases".

These comparisons clearly show that there is difficulty in nomenclature. However this distinction should not be taken too far. Clearly Christian denominations distinguish between passive euthanasia and removing futile or extraordinary or disproportionate treatment. Passive euthanasia remains wrong and is restricted to define situations in which the end has not yet been approached. Conversely Muslim scholars are in general agreement about the legitimacy of removing futile treatment and the permissibility of not given extraordinary care in order not to prolong the agony but clearly do refer to this as passive euthanasia. This is true for most Muslim countries. A global understanding of end-of-life care should therefore address this issue of nomenclature. But on the other hand, although a moral position is clear in many Christian countries, health care professionals may be more concerned with legal positions. There is less medical paternalism and patients, and their relatives can certainly challenge removal of futile care. Conversely there may be a lack of one's own moral understanding of what is licit. In all denominations therefore, families and even physicians may see removal of futile treatment or extraordinary cases as passive euthanasia and preoccupy themselves with moral and legal positions. This certainly holds as true for Christian cultures as has been seen for Muslim cultures showing the need for not only educating health care professionals but providing support and general media education to the general public and encouraging legal change.

Whilst religions may differ on whether removing extraordinary treatment is defined as passive euthanasia or not, they agree in general about its moral appropriateness. There is, however, a lack of local legislation and more modern ideas of what is commonly seen as customary in medicine may come to be more requested with people making higher demands on health care.

Pain management and sedation

The concept of pain management in many countries remains elusive. Although there is no evidence that pain management may hasten death this notion has provided moralists in many religions some thought. The Catholic religion acknowledges that even if giving pain relief can bring about an earlier death, it follow the principle of double effect in which the intention is to relieve pain and the harm is foreseen but unintended. It remains morally acceptable and is seen as a charitable thing to do. Yet lack of education in this regard entices fear in many relatives and health care professionals.

Kirchheimer (2004) argued about a decade ago that end-of-life care remains best in hospice services. In other institutions studies showed that nearly 25% did not receive adequate treatment. When considering that some patients need minimal pain relief this percentage may even be a low reflection if one had to study patients who only needed higher doses of pain relief. Thomson (2001) had also pointed out that there is a large gap between what patients desire at the end-of-life and what the system actually delivers when it comes to pain management. She quotes a survey of oncologists to said that 76% of physicians rated poor pain assessment as the single most important bar towards adequate pain management and 86% felt that patients were under-medicated. She laments the lack of attention to pain given in medical school curricula and lack of its assessment. In one study trainees show great interest in receiving training on palliative care (Mallia & Abela, 2011; Abela & Mallia, 2010)

Lack of appropriate training was reflected with the implementation and failure of the Liverpool Care Pathway (LCP) which was introduced in the UK. Whilst many British people receive end-of-life care in hospices, these, being charities, are more frequently found in the relatively richer areas of the UK. Poorer communities still were resorting to hospitalized care at the end-of-life with the result that an attempt was made to introduce palliative care in hospitals and hence the Liverpool Care Pathway. As the name implies it was a 'pathway' recommending certain steps depending on deterioration and situations. However, being a palliative care pathway, although finding itself on the National Institute of Health and Care Excellence (NICE) guidelines, it needed adequate training even of qualified doctors, which was not the case. The result was that in many places implementing the LCP meant an immediate termination of treatment, hydration and even giving sedation. It thus quickly was accused of becoming a euthanasia pathway. It was removed and new pathways were recommended to introduce adequate training (Saunders, 2013).

Very recently an article in the American Medical Association Journal of Ethics reported common misconceptions about pain management, with concerns about pain relief at the cost of some consciousness or length of life (Berger & Vadivelu, 2013) clearly showing a current lack of oral understanding and education among health care professionals. Moreover, the concept of palliative sedation gave rise to strong debate about whether this constitutes a euthanasia practice. Ten Have and Welie discussed this concept in depth in the *Journal of Pain and Symptom Management* (Ten Have & Welie, 2014). They argue that the ethical differences between palliative sedation and euthanasia are implicit. However, the concept did give rise to concerns that the practice may verge on euthanasia. They rebut this conclusion but do point out that if physicians resort immediately to sedation to circumvent existential suffering without previously trying other adequate alternatives, and also insist on removing artificial nutrition and hydration, then it will be difficult to argue that their intent is solely to relieve pain. This is in fact similar to what happened with the Liverpool Care Pathway. The International Association of Catholic Bioethics also released a statement saying that when titrated it was good practice. This makes sense as attempting to keep consciousness to give a chance to the patient to redeem himself is silly when he or she is already under the influence of drugs (Sullivan & Heng, 2013).

This concern with removing consciousness is mostly a religious concern is also reflected in Islamic practice. Many Muslim authors point out that pain is redemptive but have still concluded that end-of-life removal of pain is still consistent with Islamic teachings. Zahedi et al. (2007) argue that "pain functions as an instrument in revealing God's purpose for humanity and in reminding us that ultimately we belong, and will return to, God." They assert however that according to 'some' Muslim scholars, patients in pain from terminal illness may receive pain management. Sachedina (2005) is more optimistic in his analysis. He too asserts the same function of pain in God's plan but says that this religious and spiritual assessment of pain does not remove the fact that the primary obligation of the physician is to remove pain. This notwithstanding, many Muslims resign themselves to pain as they believe it purifies them and that pain should therefore be endured with patience and persistence. These religious purposes find their ways in both religious denominations and yet both speak about the usefulness of recognizing that pain management is important at the end-of-life and that it is not immoral practice even if it shortens life or removes consciousness.

AtiGhetchi (2007) points out that doctors in Riyadh complained about the lack of moral awareness in there country and advocated against the fear that the use of opioid analgesics goes against Islamic principles and recommended the instruction of religious authorities in order to include them in the palliative care staff. He notes the fear in many countries to resort to opioid management: in Egypt the use of morphine requires the authority of the Ministry of Health and the pharmaceutical companies and chemists prefer not to deal with morphine out of fear of the responsibility involved. In Indonesia recourse is made to non-steroidal and non-opioids and at most weak opioids due to the lack of morphine.

In the UAE, Abuhasna and Ali Abdulkareem (2013, p. 251) point out that symposiums and conferences have been addressing the need of adequate palliative care and other end-of-life issues. They are optimistic that there is a growing understanding for the need of a federal policy on dealing with terminally ill patients. They assert that interpreting the Qur'an shows that pain relief and sedation do not fall within the scope of euthanasia. Bagheri (2013, p. 279) also notes this interpretation of the Qur'an, agreeing with Sachedina that (as in the Christian tradition) that there are two situations which although interpreted as passive euthanasia are nevertheless allowed morally – palliative pain relief and removal of extraordinary treatment.

Cautionary reflections on humanists

This paper has focused on a reflection and comparison of Islamic and Christian formal thoughts on end-of-life care. Admittedly needs to analyze this comparison on a broader aspects to include other religions, especially the other important monotheistic religion of Judaism. This limit is acknowledged and hopefully the future will hold further comparison to harmonize health care. However, this paper will not be complete without a small caution on humanists. Over ten years ago, when *The Lancet* produced a series of articles on end-of-life, the humanist point of view was also discussed. Humanists are those people who consider themselves atheists but who still have concern about a moral life. They may not believe in after-life, but they have strong moral values. Of importance is that it is a Western tradition of religious thought. It is of importance here because many humanists may indeed come from families with religious backgrounds but who along the course of their lives rejected religious authority and beliefs. However one may argue that humanist inherit moral values from a western tradition. Although humanists have been traced back to ancient Greek times, their moral roots are found in the enlightenment. Certainly, although rejecting many religious belief, they positively embrace moral rules which built western moral thought. Humanists are not those people who believe in New Age, spiritualism, eastern religions or even embrace a belief in reincarnation. A prerequisite of a humanist is that they do not embrace any form of the supernatural.

The important point however is that they do believe and need propoer end-of-life care. Baggini and Pym point out that they often need to talk about their death. Death is difficult for them and their families too. Whilst one should not consider that religion can do them no harm, and therefore impose some last-minute confession or last rites, it does not follow that they do not have an interest in what happens after their death. They will be interested in the way they are buried, for example, and what we say about them. One cannot assume that because some people do not have religious beliefs, then they have fewer needs than those who do believe. One must take care that these needs are met and a discussion on harmonization at the end-of-life would be futile without considering those among us who do not share the same belief but who still have moral values. Whilst some of them may believe in euthanasia, others do not necessarily do so and the same values described here ought to be discussed with particular attention.

Conclusion

It is clear that both the Islamic and Christian religions are in agreement on positions of futile treatments, the appropriate distinction between ordinary and extraordinary care and in fact the difference between killing and allowing one to die. There is also general moral agreement on palliative pain relief and to a certain extent on sedation. None of these would be considered euthanasia. There is however some inconsistency in terminology. Whilst Christian denominations distinguish between passive euthanasia (which remain wrong) and the appropriateness of the above practices, Muslim traditions continue to refer to them as (permissible) instances of passive euthanasia. However one notices also similar fears of use owing to both the lack of legislation and perhaps fear of improper moral practices.

Conversely patients or their families in both religions often assert their rights to extraordinary care; sometimes to keep the patient alive and at others because they may believe that not providing such care is a moral practice which is disallowed. There is thus continued need for public education, legislation and indeed the support and training of health care professionals and spiritual people who may come in touch with dying people. End-of-life care is a pseudo-specialty and although palliative care is a specialist area in many western countries most patients at the end-of-life dying in hospital may not receive such specialized attention. Indeed whether it should be a specialty in its own right or a sub-specialty to be given as training in many other specialists – internal medicine, surgery, geriatrics family medicine etc. could be the subject of another analysis. With the impact of globalization, the harmonization of end-of-life care is as important as the harmonization of general medical care. A comparison of religious moral theories is important notwithstanding the secularization in many countries. The same countries often deal with people of different cultures and respecting these cultures is important to families and patients. Bringing this bioethics to the people via further studies, education and legislation is the scope of improving *clinical* outcomes and ethics.

References

Abela, J. & Mallia, P. 2010, "An evaluation of palliative care education in the specialist training programme in family medicine", *Malta Medical Journal,* vol. 22, no. 04, pp. 26-26-33.

Abuhasna, S. & Abdulkareem Al Obaidli, A. 2013, "Medical Futility in the United Arab Emirates" in *Medical Futility. A Cross-National Study*, ed. A. Bagheri, Imperial College Press, London, New Jersey, pp. 247-247-261.

Archdiocese of Atlanta 1990, "*Giorgia man asks to turn off life-supporting ventilator*" in *Quality of Life. The New Medical dilemma*, ed. James J. Walter, Thomas A. Shannon, Paulist Press, New York and Mahwah, pp. 349-357.

Arda, B., & Aciduman, A. 2013, "Medical Futility in Turkey" in *Medical Futility. A Cross-National Study*, ed. A. Bagheri, Imperial College Press, London, New Jersey, pp. 227-227-245.

AtiGhetchi, D. 2007, *Islamic Bioethics: Problems and Perspectives,* Springer, Dorthrecht.

Bagheri, A. 2013, "Medical Futility in Iran" in *Medical Futility. A Cross-National Study*, ed. A. Bagheri, Imperial College Press, London, New Jersey, pp. 263-263-282.

Ballatt, J., & Campling, P. 2013, *Intelligent Kindness. Reforming the culture of health care.* RCPsych Publications, London.

Berger, J.M. & Vadivelu, N. 2013, "Common misconceptions about opioid use for pain management at the end-of-life", *AMA Journal of Ethics,* vol. 15, no. 5, pp. 403-403-409.

Bynum, W.F. & Porter, R. (eds) 2001, *Companion Encyclopaedia of the History of Medicine, Vol. 2*, Routledge, London, New York.

Engelhardt, H.T. & Smith Iltis, A. 2005, "End-of-Life: the traditional Christian view", *The Lancet,* vol. 366, pp. 1045 - 1049.

Howard, P. & Bogle, J. 2005, *Medical Law and Ethics,* Blackwell Publishing, USA, UK, Australia.

Hinton, J. 1967, *Dying,* Penguin Books.

Kirchheimer, S. 2004, *End-of-life care inadequate, Jan 6, 2004.* Available: http://www.webmd.com/healthy-aging/news/20040106/end-of-life-care-inadequate [2015, Jan 6, 2004].

Magisterium of the Catholic Church 1994, *Catechism of the Catholic Church,* Veritas, Dublin, Vatican City.

Mallia, P. 2015, *EndCare. On Harmonization and Dissemination of Good Practice at the End-of-Life. Project no. 2015-1-MT01-KA203-003728.*

Mallia, P. & Abela, J. 2011, "An evaluation of the Palliative Care Module in the Specialist Training Programme in Family Medicine", *Malta Medical Journal,* vol. 22, no. 4, pp. 26-33.

Markwell, H. 2005, "End-of-Life: a Catholic view", *The Lancet,* vol. 366, pp. 1132 - 1135.

Miller, T.S. 1997, *The birth of the Hospital in the Byzantine Empire,* The Johns Hopkins University Press, Baltimore and London.

Pellegrino, E.D. 2009, "Toward a virtue-based normative ethics for the health professions", *Kennedy Institute of Ethics journal,* vol. 5, no. 3, pp. 253-277.

Petrini, M. 2011, "Il testamento biologico: status of art.", *Um. Nuova,* vol. 6, no. 198, pp. 621-657.

Sachedina, A. 2005, "End-of-Life: the Islamic view", *Lancet,* vol. 366, pp. 774-779.

Saunders, J. 2013, "The Liverpool Care Pathway", *Journal of the Malta College of Family Doctors,* vol. 2, no. 2, pp. 5-5-10.

Shannon, T.A. & Kockler, N.J. 2009, *An Introduction to Bioethics,* 4th edn, Pauline Press, New Jersey.

Sullivan, D. & Heng, J. 2013, "The use of sedatives in the care of persons who are seriously ill or dying. Ethical distinctions and practical recommendations. The fifth international Association of Catholic Bioethicists.", *Bioethics Outlook,* vol. 24, no. 2.

Ten Have, H. & Welie, J. 2014, "Palliative Sedation versus Euthanasia: An Ethical Assessment", *Journal of Pain and Symptom Management,* vol. 47, no. 1, pp. 123-123-136.

Thomson, H. 2001, "A new law to improve pain management and end-of-life care", *Western journal of Medicine,* vol. 174, no. 3, pp. 161-161-162.

Tillett, G. 2002, *Resolving Conflict. A practical approach,* 2nd edn, Oxford University Press, Oxford, New York.

United States Conference of Catholic Bishops 2009, *Ethical and religious directives for Catholic health care services*, 5th edn, USA.

Veatch, R.M. 2013, "So-called Futile Care: The Experience of the United States" in *Medical Futility. A Cross-National Study,* ed. A. Bagheri, Imperial College Press, London, New Jersey, pp. 9-9-33.

Walker, P. & Lovat, T. 2015, "Concepts of personhood and autonomoy as they apply to end-of-life decisions in intensive care", *Medicine, Health Care and Philosophy*, vol. 18, no. 3, pp. 309-309-315.

Zahedi, F., Larijani, B. & Tavakoly Bazzaz, J. 2007, "End-of-life ethical issues and Islamic views", *Iran Journal of Allergy Astham and Immunology*, vol. 6, no. 5, pp. 5-5-15.

Chapter 12
Palliative care for elderly – it's not only about cancer

In western societies aging has become associated with dying (Mackinlay, 2012). However the elderly are living more now and politicians and social scientists worry about the increasing proportion of the elderly population with the working one. Moreover people are having less children to the point that governments have started to encourage families to have more. The increase in opportunities for work is shown by how many people from different regions of the world are given working permits in Europe. That the elderly live longer is a good thing but one has also to look not only at the quality of life that they have, rather than spending ten years in a room doing nothing, but also the decreased opportunities for them to live alone and to be visited by their family, who may live far away or indeed unable to see them on a daily basis when they do not.

We have to admit that it is only right that we treat the elderly and give them a longer life. However we also have to enter into conversation with them about their quality of life and see what *the individual* actually wants. Whilst one patient in a home with multiple pelvic and hip fractures and blindness (and also with diabetes and hypertension) lives an active life walking marathons for a local charity), others who are in bed feel that their family have let them down and are depressed. The issue is difficult to tackle; it is like asking someone whether they want to live a shorter active life or a longer but inactive and perhaps lonely one. As one never knows what the future holds it is not as easy as when discussing Advance Care Planning for those who have cancer or a terminal disease. Having said that family doctors, and nurses, including those working in homes for elderly person can detect opportunities when someone makes a statement like, "Why has God not taken me yet", by being *trained* on how to respond with questions which allow the person to think through it and discuss with the family. Not easy but morally safe in order to find out whether the person simply wishes to be left alone or be given active treatment to prolong one's life. It should be pointed out that one is not speaking about euthanasia but simply whether one would want to be on some of the medication they have been on for decades and not providing any symptomatic relief, or, for example, whether they would want CPR. Conversely if one gets a hypoglycaemic attack, one should obviously treat as not doing so would be active euthanasia. Hypoglycaemia is a symptom and side effect of the illness at the same time at this age.

What is palliative care for the elderly

So, what is Palliative Care and what does it mean for the elderly? "Palliative Care affirms life and regards dying as a normal process. In recognising this, palliative care neither hastens nor postpones death; it helps people relief from pain and suffering and offers support to the person and his or her family" (Mackinlay, 2012). The same author points out, as doctors know only too well, that the elderly do not necessarily have a terminal illness. Many suffer with chronic heart disease, diabetes, hypertension, chronic lung disease, and dementia also become much more common in later life. All this simply because people are living longer. We have done a good job. But we have to be prudent and moderate and not simply seek to prolong or to shorten life. The balance needs to be discussed in professional development and subsequently with the person and the family if necessary. Most elderly people die from their chronic disease and it is only then that 'normal' palliative care nowadays jumps in – such as relieving shortness of breath or pain.

We need to define what a palliative care strategy or the elderly means and consists of. Hospice is a palliative care for those with cancer, especially as they approach the end-of-life. It is well organised, and a lot of experience has been obtained. At some stage the awareness and recognition of impending death does and will happen. At this time the change from active treatment to palliative is very feasible.

The most common underlying causes of death in the UK aged 75 and older are:[1]

[1] Mackinley, 2012

- Cardiovascular
- Cancer
- Respiratory disease
- Other causes

To break down even further, we have:

- Chronic ischaemic heart disease – 10%
- Pneumonia (unspecified organism) – 7.4%
- Acute myocardial infarction – 6.2%
- Stroke (not specified whether haemorrhagic or infarction) – 4.7%
- Other chronic obstructive pulmonary diseases – 4.7%
- Malignant neoplasms of bronchus and lung – 4.2%
- Unspecified dementia – 4.1%
- Other cerebrovascular diseases – 2.9%
- Semility – 2.8%
- Heart failure – 2.2%

Palliative care should and ought to aim for an improving quality of life and not simply pain relief and comfort for the elderly to thrive in a way we would all wish for ourselves in the future. It is achieved through regular contact and not simply a service of cleaning rooms, distributing meals and coffee and perhaps having an activities coordinator. “It is achieved through physical, psychosocial and spiritual care”. Spiritual care has become almost anathema these days; but be that as it may many elderly have lived a of belief and many do still have the belief that “God will take care of everything”. But God works through us. Those who may not believe in God, or have their doubts, will nevertheless realise that the lives of those who are dependent depend to a large extent of life. Thankfully many do find *meaning* in their work by being joyful and communicative. This can be seen in the brightening of the faces of those encountered. There will be those elderly who are problematic and tackling this is not easy especially if they are a nuisance to others. Only those who work in homes or who care for the elderly at home know how much pressure this work involves. These people *also* need a break. An inclusive society has to aim at both ends of life. We have made locally much advances in including children, such as those with Down Syndrome[2].

[2] Incidentally many call it Down's Syndrome, but the proper name is Down Syndrome.

Finding meaning is not only about being jolly and spending time, important as these are. It is also transcending and finding support for the suffering we as carers endure both because we may feel bad for the person and also because of the trouble the person can find. Suffering can only be alleviated by dedication and kindness. It has to be an intelligent kindness where one distributes time proportionately to needs and finds space for oneself. Otherwise palliative care becomes simply a chore like passing meals around.

A culture of service

Spirituality is important when people feel depersonalised and feel helpless or fear of impending death. For those not yet at this stage spirituality is also finding meaning at this stage of life, such as the marathon man described above. Another ninety-year-old gentle finds meaning in dancing. He has been dancing since his youth and continued it as a hobby throughout his life. He finds meaning in still going to dances and also shows his 'moves' to the young carers at the home. He provides joy to himself and others. So spiritual care is not only about finding some transcendental meaning; it is about finding meaning in life. After all if we are to find true spiritual meaning it is not about prayer only, but about what we can do for ourselves and others. This applies to the elderly as well as their carers.

Mackinley continues to explore spirituality as the ultimate meaning through:

1. Relationship
- Intimacy with other and/or God
- Emotional care

2. Environment
- Nature, sea, mountains, gardens
- Is the home close to a Garden? Even cemeteries these days are being seen as places of having gardens where even young people can go
- Do we organise visit to places and allow people the right conditions to enjoy? (last two points are my additions)

3. The arts
- Music, art, dancing

4. Religion
- Worship, prayer, reading of scripture
- Meditation

Meaning in life helps people make sense of their life at this age. Old age, no matter how much we have extended it by caring for chronic diseases, continues to be life and feeling useless is the worse service to others. Mackinay, a spiritual carer herself, notes that spiritual care may not only be given by priests or nuns, but also by doctors, nurses, social workers as well as other traditional ones. We can do this also by:

1. Spontaneous visits to see how they are
2. Defining a support network and who to call in case of accident or anything else
3. Trying to keep them at home instead of suggesting they go into a home – unless of course that is what *they* want, or it is inevitable
4. Seeing that they are supported in the available services

People may experience spiritual distress and one may start with talking through the feelings if one wants to. They may also suggest a visit by someone more professional. This service locally is provided mostly by priests. But why not train older nuns and other professionals, who may be starting to understand this experience hermeneutically[3]. Even for those without a religion this 'ritual' and other symbolism is important. People may use terms like 'the universe' or others; this is synonymous in believing in something transcendental after all why give a 'mind' symbolically to the universe when one refers to it as *the* Universe, "what the universe has ready for me".

Services

Government services can become mundane; they are usually provided by contract and tenders. Meals on wheels has become a box left behind your door for many – not even a half-minute of human contact to

[3] Hermeneutics is understanding someone or something (like a book) through your own experience. We can understand what pain is more, when we have been through it. You can never really *know me* but you can understand, especially when entering into conversation.

say hello. There is no greeting and no human contact. It must mean more than just a delivery. The food may also need to be revamped occasionally; but that is another matter. The same goes with cleaning services. One elderly lady told me that the cleaning lady just comes to wash the corridor and toilet and perhaps the kitchen floor. This is fine, but can it not be a more meaningful service in which the person engages in conversation with the woman who is alone most of the day.

We need to create a culture of service – and a service which refuses 'tips' which range from 5 euro up to 20 euro. This is a stain on our society. One nurse in one of our homes-for-elderly even condoned it with a resident stating, 'why not?' Well, the answer is obvious – one gives a preference to those who 'pay' you. It is either a free service or a paying one. Paying ones become more about the money and one will again tend to look at one's watch and get on with it to earn the next cash-in-hand. Those who do not have the money will end up just having the corridors washed.

If this is all wishful thinking, we should really consider that these services be run by voluntary institutions – from Churches to liberal groups who may honestly want to change the world. But first we must keep our own house in order before we ask the rest of the world to keep theirs'.

Providing a *good* service means providing also the human element of greeting, enjoying a small conversation and not rushing through the process from house to house or doing it merely for money. We continue as elderly to find meaning, purpose and hope through human services – we feel validated. Elderly need to have someone to communicate with and this is a services which until now is provided only as a paying one. Elderly need to be able to speak freely, to recount stories of their lives, to discuss and process problems or lack of achievement, to feel accepted, loved and approved by other and even by God for all their failures. They need to know they are preparing for death, at least subconsciously, or in the back of their minds.

Our life story is important. Elderly recount their lives for a reason. They repeat and repeat it perhaps not knowing why. But the human is a Story-telling animal (if one may be allowed to use this term) – even biologically. Psychologically there is a reason which has been less studied. We unfold our stories because we want to relate, to be understood, to reconcile, and perhaps to be remembered for what we have done, for who are and who we were at our prime. Recently I read the foreword to a book on a local politician. The author said it was a very good biography, but added, something to the effect like "not like the many biographies we see on sale of people (hardly known) who have only done their duty". He basically said that they have nothing to say. But everyone has something to say and we may not all have the life-story to have a 'good' biography worth buying. We often buy biographies of our heroes – politicians, film stars, footballers, etc. But if we could have for posterity a free biographical service in whatever form, recorded, written, formal or informal, as some commendable television programmes are doing, we will have material to inspire future generations and see the life people lives, especially in this day and age where future generations have become an issue for international bodies, especially with climate change, uncontrolled industry, consumerism, artificial intelligence, robots, neurotechnology, and so on.

If the service provider gets meaning in their life, then they are providing a source of meaning to the person served. Being their server does not mean being their servant – as the film said. There are hopes, joys, disappointments, adventures, achievements and so much more to many people's lives. After all it is not only the popular actors or sports persons who have something to say. They were blessed with something which is popular. But their personal lives may be quite different than what we imagine and frought with pride, drugs and tragic deaths. They do indeed have something to say as well. But just because we are not popular does not mean we do not have something we wish, may, or perhaps more important, ought to pass along. As the Maltese saying goes, '*kliem ix-xiħ żomm fih*' – as well as '*ix-xiħa*'. They may not agree with the modern way of life, but they still have something worth saying. You see an unkempt old lady in a dirty home and very disabled due to chronic disease, and yet one would be surprised, if only one befriended them, to know what they have to say. This has been my experience as a family doctor (general practitioner), and I regret when either out of not having the time or for some other reason, I did not spend so much time with one of our elderly. Moreover, I have been nourished and learned considerably by experiences in which I put aside the time to listen to. These people need only give a word of advice and having known them I usually take it. We all have time to learn through our services.

References

Mackinley E., *Palliative Care, Aging and Spirituality – a guide for older people, carers, and families*, Jessica Kingsley Publishers, London and Philadelphia, 2012

Further reading

Kerr, D., Wilkinson, H., *Providing Good Care at Night for Older People – practical approaches for use in nursing and care homes*, Jessica Kingsley Publishers, London and Philadelphia, 2011

Lee, E., *In Your Own Time – a guide for patients and their carers facing a last illness at home*, Oxford University Press, Oxford, 2002.

Formosa, M. (ed.), *Active and Health Ageing in Malta – gerontological and geriatric inquiries*, BDL Publishing, 2018.

Chapter 13
Consensus document with guidelines on end-of-life care[1]

Preface from coordinator of the project

The End Care Project started with the realisation that end-of-life care is not homogenous notwithstanding that we have ample moral sources to harmonise it. End-of-life care has become medicalised. Many have come to expect nothing less than miraculous cures even when people suddenly approach an unexpected death. A consultant recently told me that when faced with a patient who was dying a discussion arose with one of his registrars who had come from the UK and who had suggested the Liverpool Care Pathway, which was intended to be nothing more than a Palliative Care pathway for the dying and accepted in the NICE guidelines. The consultant replied that in Malta euthanasia is not accepted. One cannot blame him as the LCP turned out not to be applied with proper training and became a tick-box where all people who were put on the pathways suddenly had all treatment, hydration and nutrition stopped. This of course was a misapplication, as all know, of the pathway and led to the 'One chance to get it right' document. It was a learning experience. People were simply abandoned on a 'pathway' which was meant to provide them with proper end-of-life care as was done in Hospices throughout the UK. The pathway was developed for those people who did not have access to hospices. It turned out not to have been practiced as a pathway.

[1] Faculty Of Medicine & Surgery, Faculty of Laws, Faculty Of Theology
Bioethics Research Programme and Medicine & Law Programme
As part of an Erasmus+ project of the Bioethics Research Programme of the Medical School, on Harmonisation of end-of-life care (EndCare)
University of Malta
Endorsed by: The National Bioethics Consultative Committee
Compiled by Professor Pierre Mallia (Coordinator of the Erasmus+ EndCare Project, https://www.um.edu.mt/r/projects/endcare)

Countless books written by doctors exist on the discontent the profession feels about the incoherent way we treat dying people. Ought we to keep them alive as much as possible? When ought we to stop nutrition and even hydration? When is it a discomfort? Many have the conviction that we should at least provide hydration. And indeed most people dying in hospital do so with a drip attached to them. Yet when someone dies at home it is accepted that this is not always possible. Is hydration a part of dying naturally? Does it really provide the comfort we think it does? Are we convinced that a doctor on call who is asked to change a drip on a dying patient ought to puncture the patient a number of times trying to find a vein which is not collapsed? Are we convinced that these patients do not feel that pain? Who makes the call to stop hydration nowadays? Even when we stop nutrition, doctors and nurses may disagree with other health care professionals who may insist on nutrition via a PEG. These people will eventually need to evacuate their bowel. But do dying people need nutrition in their last days? Most people who die naturally do so without food. It is appropriate in conscious or semiconscious, no doubt. But it is a fact that we may not be preparing patients and relatives and indeed ourselves that dying people to not need nutrition and that this may simply be prolonging the agony. As the GMC guidelines recommend, we need to recognise the imminence of death and move towards a plan so as not to come towards the end with doubts on whether to increase morphine due to the fear of respiratory suppression to even whether re-inserting and intravenous line to provide fluids is necessary when we are expecting the patient to die very soon.

This document is a result of the EndCare Erasmus+ project of the Bioethics Research Programme in the Faculty of Medicine & Surgery, Mater Dei Hospital. Preliminary studies we carried out did show that many doctors are concerned about legal issues and lack of understanding of relatives of what *ought* to be done. Therefore we resort to what *can* be done. It is with this understanding that this project involved not only the Faculty of Medicine and Surgery of the University of Malta but also the Faculties of Laws and of Theology; the former to give us the legal guidance, the lack of which was complained about and the latter to remind us of the accepted moral practice. The EndCare (Erasmus+) project also partnered with Dublin

City University and the University of L'Aquila, besides experts from law, philosophy, theology, bioethics and institutions like UNESCO and the Pontifical Academy for Life of the Vatican.

There is a sea between theoretical bioethics, which gives us the necessary grounding of our moral actions, and clinical ethics when one is faced with a real patient and real relative; and not least a team which not only wants to do well by the patient but want to *be seen* to be doing what is just.

It is hoped that this document will be accepted by the Medical Council. It has been highly commended by the Minister for health who is concerned about legal issues as much as all doctors are. It is fine to follow moral guidance which is even found in sections of death and dying in the Catholic Catechism; but it is another thing not to be sure that the law is behind you and that you are not in danger of stopping treatment which is futile or which the patient considered to be extraordinary. The document has to ideally also be read by the other material of the project which includes a detailed curriculum for retreats and summer schools and recommendations of Advanced Care Planning (to be distinguished from legally-binding documents such as Advanced Directives which can sometimes cause more dilemmas).

Advanced Care Planning already happens to a certain extend by general practitioners when people decide to die at home. We discuss what is available and what is not. Family doctors know when to stop treatment because they explain its futility in the presence of relatives and at a time convenient to them. They speak with relatives and explain when 'time has come'. *But they are at an advantage.* The general practitioner has known the family for quite some time; there is a fiduciary relationship built over years. It is not the same in a hospital where personnel change according to a time table and decision made perhaps only during ward rounds and where ideas can vary on whether we should keep that drip, even at least subcutaneously.

The frustration of many health professionals and the input of many of them has led to this local document which one hopes will be followed by the necessary retreats/summer schools necessary. The summer school we help in 2016 was a success and attended by nurses, doctors (not least consultants working with dying patients), and paramedical professionals. The recent debate on euthanasia showed that those who agreed with made statements like, "why should one die in pain" or "why should one be put on a machine that she/he does not want". One of our Master's thesis in Clinical Ethics & Law brought out the important finding that nurses do not see as morally equivalent withholding treatment and withdrawing of treatment. The latter is more emotionally charged, indeed, but it should not be feared. We hope that this document alleviates these concerns and brings people together to discuss end-of-life.

Last but not least we tackle Spirituality – a subject which should not be left to the priest alone. We all need to contribute. Spirituality is finding meaning in one's existence towards the end-of-life. It is a conversation with people. I thank therefore the Faculty of Theology and the Faculty of Laws and those involved who have helped with this document. Just as philosophy is driven by scientific knowledge, so should science be driven by philosophical and ethical reflection and guidance. This has led to proper laws and amendments. Medicine is the field which brings all life experience, from science to philosophy and law together. No wonder it has been called an art. To this art at the end-of-life we must reflect so as to move away from what has become a medicalization of death, simply because home deaths have decreased because of changing family dynamics and social life.

I sincerely hope that this is only the beginning of the process and that the document can serve as a comfort to those who know what they ought to do but find the necessary framework insufficient. It is with pleasure that the Hon. Deputy Prime Minister and Minister for Health, Mr Chris Fearne has invited me to present this document to officials in the Ministry and the Department of Health and he is to invite me to address parliamentarians to effect any necessary changes in the law. I can only conclude by thanking him for the interest he has taken not only in this project but in clinical ethics in hospital and in general.

Professor Pierre Mallia
Coordinator, EndCare Erasmus+, and the Bioethics Research Programme,
University of Malta, Msida, 26th February 2018

The following three messages were forewords to the original document:

Word by the dean of the Faculty of Medicine & Surgery

The Bioethics Research Programme (BRP) has recognised the importance of end-of-life care and the problems both locally and internationally this has brought with it. Medicalization of death has indeed become an issue as many medical journals are now attesting. The concept of the study in fact started with a seminar on end-of-life organised by the same Programme which took place during the controversy of the Liverpool Care Pathway whilst at the same time many of our consultant were contracting the BRP coordinator for advice. EndCare is an Erasmus+ project which was awarded almost half a million euros and coordinated by our Faculty. It has produced some good results, one of which is this guidance for health care professionals, especially doctors, in collaboration with the Faculty of Laws and the Faculty of Theology. We would like to thank the Deans of these Faculties, Prof. Kevin Aquilina and Prof. Emanuel Agius for their support and help in reviewing the general guidance for legal and moral issues respectively.

It is hoped that with the guidance our medical staff will find comfort in the support and advice it provides. The BRP has followed Maltese law and the General Medical Council guidelines of the UK, adapting it to our local needs. I commend the Bioethics Research Programme for the work and energy it has put into end-of-life care and this project. Indeed the project had three summer schools, one in Malta, one in L'Aquila Italy, and one in Dublin, where our project partners are. We have had the guidance of experts from UNESCO, UK, France, and indeed the Pontifical Academy for Life. The summer schools were very informative and successful and this guidance will also serve as material for future summer school to be held in Malta which will also have the backing of Erasmus and the University of Malta.

Professor Godfrey La Ferla
Dean, Faculty of Medicine & Surgery,
University of MaltaMsida, 26th February 2018

Word by the dean of the Faculty of Laws

As Dean of the Faculty of Laws at the University of Malta it gives me pleasure to write a short Foreword to this Consensus Statement. The latter has been drawn up by the Faculties of Medicine and Surgery, Laws and Theology, with the active participation of the Bioethics Research Programme and the Medicine and the Law Programmes of the University of Malta. I remain indebted to the collaboration received from the Government of Malta's National Bioethics Consultative Committee and the Medical Council of Malta.

This Consensus Statement is the result of an Erasmus+ project of the Bioethics Research Programme of the Medical School on *Harmonisation of end-of-life care (EndCare)* which has brought together representatives from the entities listed in the first paragraph and international scholars who have produced a much needed document intended to fill in a lacuna in Malta in relation of end-of-life care. Malta is indeed being affected by the discussion on end-of-life issues but the main problem in this field is the lack of a elaborate legislative framework to regulate end-of-life issues. But the problem is not only legal. Guidance is required also both at a moral and religious perspective in so far as end-of-life issues raise serious moral and religious considerations which cannot be dismissed. On the contrary, all these issues need to be brought together, discussed and a way forward proposed. This is essentially what this Consensus Statement does in so far as end-of-life care is concerned. It is also good to note that the principal actors in this field have come together to rack their brains and produce a document agreeable to all discussing the main areas needing direction in the realm of end-of-life care.

The Consensus Statement is of course not a law but a set of guidelines. Currently, there is a dearth of such guidance and the Consensus Statement is the first step in providing clear guidance to health care professionals who, in the exercise of their profession, are faced with apparently complex and irresolvable dilemmas which need instantaneous settlement. Hopefully it will be worked out, at a later stage, into an enactment to provide more certainty to stakeholders involved which include not only the legal and healthcare professions but also bioethicists, hospital administrators, patients and the latter's relatives. All should know where they stand on these issues and the State should provide such definitiveness. It is augured that the Medical

Council will discuss in depth these guidelines and, if need be, pass on to improve them and that, perhaps, at a later stage, when these guidelines have been tried and tested, they are enacted into law which such modifications required following the appraisal of the implementation of these guidelines.

Professor Kevin Aquilina
Dean, Faculty of Laws,
University of Malta, Msida, 19th December 2017

Word by dean of Faculty of Theology

Recent surveys carried out by the Council of Europe in its Member States reveal that end-of-life issues are gaining more and more prominence in social media debates and in public policies. As medical knowledge and technology increase, people from all walks of life are becoming more conscious and conscientious of the complex ethical dilemmas in the end-of-life decision-making process. People want an open and transparent discussion on how to resolve the psychological, spiritual, legal, existential, and medical issues surrounding end-of-life care.

Among the European institutions, the Council of Europe has been the leading fora promoting on-going debates, reports, resolution and recommendations on the dignity and rights of the terminally ill and dying patients. The Parliamentary Assembly, in its Recommendation 1418 (1999) on *Protection of the human rights and dignity of the terminally ill and the dying*, declares that the vocation of the Council of Europe is the protection of the dignity of all human beings and the rights which stem therefrom. Therefore, for the Council of Europe, it is undisputed that dealing with the concerns of the terminally ill or dying is to be guided by the notion of human dignity and the concept of human rights founded therein.

The fundamental rights of the terminally ill or dying person are threatened today by a variety of factors. Insufficient access to palliative care and good pain management; artificial prolongation of the dying process by either using disproportionate medical measures or by continuing treatment without a patient's consent; as well as the patients' fear of losing their autonomy and becoming a burden to, and totally dependent upon, their relatives or institutions are serious threats to patient's dignity and the right to be treated as a living human being until death.

The Council of Europe recommends to all member states to recognise palliative medicine and care as a legal entitlement of the individual and to ensure that relatives and friends are encouraged to accompany the terminally ill or dying and to support professionally their endeavours. Moreover, a terminally ill or dying person should receive adequate pain relief and palliative care, even if this treatment as a side-effect may contribute to the shortening of the individual's life. Furthermore, the terminally ill or dying person's expressed wishes with regard to particular forms of treatment should be taken into account, provided they do not violate human dignity.

Recommendation 1418 (1999) of the Council of Europe states unequivocally that the fundamental right to life and the prohibition of intentionally taking human life are to be upheld also under the special conditions of the terminal phase of an individual's life. Dying is a phase of life. Thus, the right to die in dignity corresponds with the right to a life in dignity. Article 2 of the *European Convention on Human Rights* declares that "no one shall be deprived of his life intentionally".

A terminally ill or dying person's wish to die never constitutes any legal claim to die at the hand of another person. In order words, a terminally ill or dying person's wish to die cannot of itself constitute a legal justification to carry out actions intended to bring about death. Taking a patient's life is no therapeutic option, since it is not directed towards terminating the patient's suffering but rather at terminating the patient himself.

Rev Professor Emmanuel Agius
Dean, Faculty of Theology,
University of Malta, Msida, 2nd March, 2018

Definitions

Advanced Care Plan: This is a *plan* which is described in detail in this document and here is *not* to be confused with Advance Directives. It is a plan which can change as the situation changes and requires only the *Capacity* (taken as defined under the Mental Health Act of Malta) and not Competence, which can be affected by one's illness.
Advance Directive: This is a legal document which a person signs before one has an illness or when an illness is diagnosed. It is drawn up by legal practitioner and must be signed by a competent person.
Disproportionate treatment: This is treatment which is no proportional to the normal standard of care in a given situation. It may be given however if there seems to be some benefit, albeit psychological or social.
Doctor: Unless otherwise stated the term refers to the consultant or physician in charge of the patient.
End-of-life: The term 'end-of-life' is used in the context of an imminence of death. The latter, as explained in the text, is taken to mean a spectrum of recognition that death will be imminent within one year up to the point where death is imminent within a few days or a few hours.
Euthanasia is taken to mean the deliberate intention to terminate the life of an individual by an act of commission (Active Euthanasia) or omission (passive Euthanasia). In this document any form of licit removal of futile treatment, treatment which is disproportionate or considered by the patient to be extraordinary are not, as in some definitions, considered as passive euthanasia. Neither is pain relief which, when provided according to a standard of due care, considered as active euthanasia if it hastens death in any way. These measures are

morally acceptable in many traditions and are considered charitable towards dying patients.

Extraordinary treatment: This is *not* futile treatment but simply treatment which may be prolonged with some benefit, albeit sometimes at some cost to the patient.

Futile treatment: Futile treatment is that treatment which is not considered by the doctor to be in any way beneficial to the patient. It is ultimately a clinical decision and is not to be confused with extraordinary or disproportionate care, which in and of themselves can provide some benefit and in which the patient ought to participate. Doctors have thus been known to stop treatment, such as inotropic agents, whilst speaking in general terms to patients and relatives that treatment will be tailed down or stopped.

Health Care Professional: (HCP) This is taken to be any professional working within the team dealing with the dying person. It includes doctors, nurses, physiotherapists, health care workers and other recognized paramedical personnel working together towards the care of patients.

Ordinary treatment or care: This is considered as the basic care required to keep a patient comfortable. One has to emphasise that the patient has to be involved as something which usually is considered as ordinary care, such as hydration, may at times be considered uncomfortable, or even disproportionate and extraordinary.

Patients' rights*:* Whenever this term is used, it is to be considered as applicable under Maltese law unless otherwise stated.

Recognition of death: This is taken to mean when one arrives to a conclusion that the patient is now dying and is expected to die within the next few hours or at most days. It is a clinical diagnosis with specified signs and symptoms.

UK: In view of developing political situations, UK is taken to mean the United Kingdom as constituted on the date of publication of this document.

Vegetative states: Although this document does not enter into a discussion of vegetative states, this term is taken to mean a neurological state which is duly diagnosed by modern equipment and is not to be confused with a Coma, or with patients who are still entering into a vegetative state. Vegetative states may be persistent or permanent.

Guidelines on end-of-life care

Introduction

The recent debate on euthanasia and end-of-life issues on the media and in public life have given rise to concern about the end-of-life processes in our homes and hospitals and indeed as to whether our traditional moral values on end-of-life are protected under Maltese law. By traditional moral values one has generally understood that one ought not to treat patients without their consent, that the patients have a right to refuse treatment and that they can choose between what they deem as ordinary care and extraordinary or disproportionate care. Conversely doctors are not obliged to give futile treatment and they can give pain relief, as long as it follows a standard of care, even if it may hasten death.

However, this does not seem to be the whole picture. Health care professionals still find it difficult to initiate discussion on end-of-life as the system seems to be geared towards cure. End-of-life is therefore not recognized when imminent and it may be difficult at that stage to discuss decisions which people may find hard to understand. Much depends on the individual carer but often there may be no coherent understanding and opinions may vary. On the media one often hears complaints that it was the pain relief that killed a loved one, especially if the death occurred only a few minutes after the morphine was given. Conversely others complain of pain.

Recent surveys carried out (Abela & Mallia, 2010; Mallia & Abela, 2011) have shown that doctors are concerned that there may not be enough protection of the law when deciding about futile treatment, that it is not clear that the patients decide about what is extraordinary care for them and indeed whether they have clear rights to refuse life-prolonging treatment. Also there is a general concern that the public does not understand the moral issues at the end-of-life, even though many follow a Christian (more often Catholic) faith. There is also a rise in people of Islamic faith. Many are not sure about the coherence and agreement about end-of-life care between these two faiths. In general it is felt that authorities should be teaching more about end-of-life rather than discuss the issue of euthanasia only. Indeed recent surveys done on local televised popular programmes which questioned people about whether euthanasia ought to be a right found that amongst those who favoured euthanasia, the main reasons were that people ought not to die in pain or to suffer. Indeed that people need not die in pain and that even if pain relief hastens death, once death is recognised as the inevitable outcome, is morally acceptable by all religions seems generally not to be understood.

This consensus document is aimed therefore at providing health care professionals with clear guidance on the moral, legal and religious perspectives on end-of-life decision-making within the local context, keeping in mind normative values whilst avoiding controversial areas. Many health professionals, patients and their relatives fear making the right decisions at the end-of-life of a patient because of fear of litigation or lack of awareness of accepted moral values. This guidance, which borrows also from the General Medical Council (UK) guidance on end-of-life (General Medical Council, 2010) in areas which are of common normative value within the Maltese context, aims to clarify the following:

- The necessity of consent on the part of the patient before any treatment is started and the right to refuse life-prolonging treatment once death is an inevitable outcome or there is danger of unduly prolonging life which results in suffering or pushes patients into the dangerous zone of persistent or permanent vegetative states
- What to do if a patient lacks capacity
- Explain the difference between killing and allowing to die
- Explain the difference between providing ordinary as opposed to extraordinary or disproportionate care
- Clarify what is meant by passive euthanasia and the acceptance of avoiding futile treatment

- Reassurance on pain relief and sedation when appropriate, following a standard of care, even if this is thought to hasten death
- To recognise when death is imminent and to accept death as an inevitable outcome so as to provide the proper dignity and attention that patients deserve without putting them through undue hardship.

These guidelines do not intend to re-invent the wheel, as it were, but follow accepted international documents and guidelines listed in the bibliography. Following the British General Medical Council guidelines, 'you must' is used for an over-riding duty or principle, and 'you should' is when an explanation is provided of how one will meet this over-riding duty, or when the duty or principle will not apply in all situations or where there are factors beyond one's control.

This document is meant to be presented to the Medical Council of Malta which will be asked to approve it as guidance for doctors and health care professionals dealing with patients who are approaching the end-of-life. By definition this means when patients are likely to die within the next 12 months. This includes those whose death is imminent (expected within hours), and, following GMC guidelines, those with:

- Advanced, progressive, incurable conditions
- General frailty and co-existing conditions that mean they are expected to die within 12 months
- Existing conditions if they are at risk of dying from a sudden acute crisis in their condition
- Life-threatening acute conditions caused by sudden catastrophic events.

Principles

The principles used here are to help professionals in their work in end-of-life and in explaining to patients and relatives the medical, moral, religious and legal obligations and to promote the values of team work and working with patients and those close to them. In particular:

1. One must give patient approaching the end-of-life the same quality of care as all other patients. Patients must be treated

with dignity, respect and compassion, as must those close to them, especially when facing difficult questions about decision-making in the care of the dying person.

2. Privacy and rights to confidentiality must be respected and also the right to spiritual care.
3. There must be no discrimination based on the patient being older, having a disability or those who understandably may be referred to as 'social cases'. It is recognised that internationally as well as perhaps locally, some of these groups have experienced inequality in getting access to health services.
4. People in the care of dying people must be aware of Chapter IV of the Constitution of Malta setting out fundamental rights and freedoms and the European Convention Act, Chapter 319 of the Laws of Malta, and its main provisions on basic rights and principles.
5. There is a presumption in favour of prolonging life following established ethical and legal principles but that however there is no absolute obligation to prolong life irrespective of the consequences to the patient and irrespective of the patient's views, if they are known.
6. One must assume that every adult patient has the capacity to make decisions about their care and treatment. The difference, which can be subtle, between obtaining a proper informed choice, which includes determining competence, and making sure that the patient has capacity will be explained, as this can lead to wrongful decision, especially in groups mentioned in '3' above – for example, it can be deduced that an elderly person may not be competent and therefore unable to give proper informed consent. Yet such a patient may still have the capacity to make a decision on the care and treatment, including the capacity to refuse life-prolonging measures.
7. If a patient's capacity is limited, one must provide all the necessary support and help to maximise their ability to understand and weigh information. When capacity is impaired the one must see who is making a decision on the patient's behalf. Decisions doctors and relatives make must ensure the overall benefit of the patient, including options not to treat. Doctors must consult

closely with relatives, especially where wishes by the patient have been expressed or even documented.

8. Under Maltese law the patient has the right to refuse treatment, whether ordinary or extraordinary. This however should be discussed clearly and with respect for information and understanding and making sure it is a voluntary choice. Competence cannot be put into question if the patient has the capacity to assimilate, retrain and give consistent feedback on information.

Decision-making models (adopted from GMC-UK)

1. In patients who have capacity
    - Doctor and patient make assessment of the patient's condition taking into account the medical history, views, experiences and knowledge.
    - Doctor uses specialised knowledge, clinical judgement and patient's views to identify the treatment and any investigations which are appropriate and likely to be of benefit. Doctors must be aware not to put pressure or in any way coerce or thwart in any way information which will lead patients not to make a voluntary choice.
    - The Patient decides whether to accept the options or refuse them.
    - If the patient asks for treatment with which the doctor, after appropriate discussion, disagrees, then explanation why it is thought not to be the clinically appropriate path must be offered. Other options may be offered including the seeking of a second opinion or legal representation.

2. In patients who lack capacity
    - Doctors must be clear on the decision they think are clinically appropriate.
    - Check if there are any legally binding documents which express the patient's wishes.
    - Check whether there is a power of attorney who can discuss further care and treatment with the patient and check whether the legal scope of the power of attorney actually

covers medical decision-making.

- Take responsibility for the treatment which will provide overall benefit to the patient when no power of attorney exists and after consulting those close to the patient and the health care team.
- One must judge the validity of any documents which the patient has made.
- If the patient has granted a power of attorney, then the doctor must give the same information which would have been given to the patient and explain the benefits, burdens, and risks of the options available. Doctors must help attorneys come to decisions which overall benefit the patient, offer support and in the same way as dealing with patients with capacity, must not put pressure on the attorney.
- As well as advising the attorney the doctor must involve those close to the patient and the health care team involved as they may be able to contribute information which is relevant.
- If no attorney is available the doctors is responsible for decisions after consulting with the health care team and those close to the patient.
- If disagreement arises one must follow the procedure for conflict resolution explained in this document.

Using the principles and models

Role of relatives, partners and those close to the patient

- People close to the patient play an important role in ensuring the patient receives high quality care in both home care and the hospital setting. These people are involved in speaking and discussing with the patient helping them to come to decisions and enabling them to communicate their wishes.
- In some cases they may have legal power to make decisions.
- It is important to acknowledge the roles and responsibilities of people close to the patient and to ensure that their needs for making decisions, whilst at the same time their need for support in this difficult time, are met.
- They may need or want information about the patient's diagnosis and the likely progression of the illness in order to

help them to provide the necessary support and care. One should check that the patient agrees with this if they have capacity; if they do not one may assume it reasonable to share relevant information and to keep them informed of progress.

- One should explain clinical issues in a way the person understands and approach distressing issues with tact.
- In considering those close to the patient who do not have legal capacity, one must be clear that their role is to advise the health care team about the patient's known or likely preferences, feelings, beliefs and values. One must be clear that they are not being asked to make decisions on behalf of the patient.

Clinical decision-making and judgements

- The bio-psycho-social needs of the patient must guide decision-making.
- Where appropriate proper guidelines must be followed (e.g. the stepping up and stepping down of pain relief).
- Early consideration to palliative care must be given.
- A second opinion on management must be sought if the doctor has limited experience of the condition, there is uncertainty on how to manage symtoms effectively, and if one is in doubt about the range of options.

Emotional difficulties

- It may be more difficult to withdraw a life-prolonging treatment than it is to withhold starting such treatment, notwithstanding the principle of moral equivalence involved. This may be the cause of emotional distress but one must not allow this to hinder one's clinical judgement and the best interests of the patient or to continue with treatment which does not have overall benefit.
- Keeping a treatment going for the sake of the family is incorrect clinical practice and judgement. Conversely emotional difficulties can lead one not to start treatment which would have some benefit. This includes, but is not limited to, pain relief, which can indeed hasten death. (One must assess, for

example, what benefit one is obtaining from a hydration drip which needs replacement when knowing it will be difficult to find a vein and that the likelihood of dehydration is small. One must not assume that without a drip a patient is left dehydrated).

- One should make sure that the patient does not feel pressured into accepting or refusing particular investigations and treatments, and that they are given the time and information necessary to help them reach their own decisions.
- In this regard all the support, counselling and spiritual services must be offered, including any ethics consultations.
- One must never withdraw or not start treatment because of resource constraints. This also (and especially) includes sending people to die at home because of lack of beds notwithstanding the prerogatives that the beds can be used for other patients. It is inappropriate to breach the fiduciary relationship that exists between patients and health professionals at the end of one's life because of reasons outside the scope of the best interests of the patient.
- One must weigh the benefits and risks of treatment options. Treatment which can prolong life can also increase risks and burdens on patients. Such extraordinary or disproportionate treatment need not be given. In the end it is the patient who decides whether a treatment is extraordinary as this takes into account the patient's circumstances.
- One should explain all the options available to patients and avoid bias by withholding information because of certain circumstances, such as the difficulty a patient may find in communicating. All reasonable steps to maximise the patients' capacity must be taken.

Conflict resolution

"By its very nature the arena of medical ethics is replete with conflict. Here principle meets practical: the burden of allotting limited resources challenges what may be a morally correct course of action; personal encounters policy; a hospital-wide procedure may not fit the unique circumstances of a particular patient; and a mixed multitude, sometimes a whole committee, ponders a question ultimately in the domain of the individual. In a health care setting, doctrines of justice and patients' rights translate into concrete decisions based on immediate reality. Although an action may directly affect one particular patient, many people affect and are affected by it, and this may claim a secondary stake in what happens. Herein lies the ingredients of conflict" (Neveloff Dubler, 2005)

The principles recommended are:

1. Legal advice should be the last option
2. It is important to distinguish between a conflict and a dispute. Both involve disagreement but a conflict involves values, whereas a dispute involves disagreements which can be more easily understood.
3. One should aim to reach a consensus through mediation (see below)
4. Patients may feel that certain treatments, or mission of treatment, may go against their religious beliefs. Whilst this shows the importance of discussing options ahead of time, it also raises the issue that many may not be aware what their religion, for example, allows or disallows. This has led to misconceptions about such issues as pain relief and removal of futile treatment. Having an advanced care plan can help in resolving these issues ahead of time.
5. It is important to realise that
   - One cannot treat without the patient's consent
   - There is a difference between killing and allowing someone to die when death is the inevitable outcome
   - One can give appropriate pain relief and if necessary even sedation, even if these shorten life
   - One need not give disproportionate or futile treatment, or treatment which is considered extraordinary, especially by the patient.
6. People may be afraid that high doses of pain relief which may shorten life are active euthanasia, or, that removing a treatment which is extraordinary, disproportionate or even futile, is a form of passive euthanasia. In this case one needs to explain that there is no conflict of values about deliberately bringing about, directly or indirectly, the death of the patient.

7. One should make an effort to understand whether patients or those close to them are asking for, or refusing, a treatment or procedure because they feel it goes against their religious beliefs or that one is offering a deliberate intention to shorten life. If one is convinced that there is no clear understanding of points in 5(a-d) then one has a disagreement which is not based on value of life. One should explain that the issue may be clarified by offering the person to speak with a spiritual or ethics counsellor.
8. Families may conversely request measures which go beyond normal medical wisdom, or even make requests which are unreasonable, such as keeping someone on a life support system when there is not hope for improvement or when there is already a diagnosis of brain death.
9. Some patients or relatives may feel that certain treatment is not being provided because of cost containment or because of scarce resources. This indeed will amount to a conflict as it involves a value.
10. Clear communication is the key to effective conflict resolution

Keep in mind the following myths about conflict: (Marshall & Robson, 2018):

- Conflict can be avoided
- Conflict is bad
- Conflict is impossible to resolve
- A lawyer is always needed
- All disagreements can escalate into conflict

The origin of conflict is often due to:

- Unmet needs (including emotional)
- Lack of effective communication
- Emotional and moral distress
- Disparity of knowledge, power and control

11. Mediation is the most important and efficient route to resolving conflict, especially where there are differences in the cultures of patients, families, and health providers. One has to keep in mind that bioethical analysis favour the academic positions

which often favour the medical culture. Mediation strives to dissociate itself from closed systems of analysis and intelligence for unarticulated values and preferences of the particular patient (Neveroff Dubler, 2005).

12. Mediation may have to involve an ethicist who will:
    - Identify the parties to the conflict
    - Understand the stated and latent interests of the parties
    - Level the playing field to minimise disparities of power, knowledge, skill, and experience
    - Search for common ground, especially one that is time-sensitive
    - Ensure that the consensus reached is a 'principled resolution' in light of legal rights and ethical scholarship
    - Follow up to be sure that the agreement reached has sufficient structural support to become the reality of care (Neveroff Dubler, 2005).

Advanced Care Plans

The concept of a legally binding Advance Directive has caused concern with theoretical issues that they may be binding even if the patient or the person with legitimate power of attorney, may not make decisions which even the health professionals taking care of the patient would agree with and which they will be bound not to be able to implement.

This consensus statement therefore does not discuss Advance Directives in the contemporary traditional meaning as this would require legal implementation. It does however support the concept of an Advanced Care Plan. Although some people may use the two terms interchangeably and an Advance Care Plan will still need legal support, this can be done with existing legislation. An Advance Care Plan is decided in advance with the health care team for such a time when the patient cannot make informed choices but still has capacity (as defined in this document) or when the patient loses consciousness, allows those close to the patient to be able to discuss medical care. Although not legally binding it will provide a guide as to the patient's wishes.

It must be understood that:

1. The limits and contents of an advanced plan should remain within the law and within the contents of this document. It does not allow requests which are illegal or verge into dangerous areas. It is therefore debateable whether a patient can refuse artificial nutrition and hydration when this is not providing discomfort and when death is not yet imminent. Although one can make a case for this right to refusal, especially if invasive methods are used, this has to satisfy all concerned that the reason is not to deliberately shorten life but because the patient has been recognised to be dying and the nutrition and hydration are being refused on a basis of discomfort and that they will not provide appropriate care.
2. Conversely patients can refuse life-prolonging treatment in terminal diseases, such as motor neuron disease and if he or she considers this treatment to be extraordinary and although prolongs life, will provide a life of discomfort, pain and dependency which are unacceptable to the dignity of the patient. There have been enough international cases, decided even within religious contexts, of this possibility.
3. Doctors and health professional cannot provide any form of treatment without the patient's consent, especially if they have expressed this wish repeatedly beforehand, knowing that there will come a time when a treatment considered extraordinary would not be wanted.
4. In this circumstance the consultant must have the final say but must take into consideration the rights of the patient. Over-riding these right will be verging also into dangerous legal and moral territory which will require over-riding justifications, sometimes difficult to prove, especially when family disagree.
5. In this circumstance the consultant, when such a time as the considered extraordinary or disproportionate treatment need to be provided in order to prolong life, must:
   - Consult with the patient once again.
   - Consults the family about the wish of the family.
   - Has a right to make a consultation with another consultant or hospital ethicist.

- Must provide the patient with the necessary medical treatment so as not to allow suffering (such as sedation) or physiological distress, and accept that the patient dies a natural death whilst continuing to provide ordinary care and comfort.
- Everyone concerned must accept that what is being omitted is disproportionate and extraordinary care, which although may prolong life indefinitely, is not being given to respect the rights of the patient.
- In the absence of legal protection the consultant can have a right to an objection of conscience.
- In this case the consultant should ideally discuss this early and not when the time for the said treatment arrives, in order to find another consultant who is willing to undertake such care.

6. There is a need to formalise such requests on a document or in the patient's file. Patients should also be handed a copy which can be shown to doctors in the future.
7. It is recommended that if the refusal of treatment is controversial, such as refusing to be put on a respirator when still conscious, then the document should be countersigned by the legal representative of the patient (an attorney).
8. It should be understood that the moral is that doctors have the necessary knowledge to appraise the patient's situation from a medical point of view. They have a prime role in decision-making; but it is recognised that rights and social issues must be balanced from case to case.
9. Refusal of a particular treatment means ONLY removal of that treatment. As with a DNACPR order, it refers only to that procedure and NOT to other treatments.
10. This should be communicated well among the team looking after the patient and the patient should not be labelled as having had all treatment stopped. With proper care and comfort, and if necessary treatment not yet considered futile, patients may continue to live for a number of days comfortably. One is simply respecting the right to refuse a procedure which is considered disproportionate and extraordinary, albeit not futile, by the patient.

11. Ultimately, the decision-making process should be the result of:
    - *Information* The patients and relatives have to understand the concepts well and social institutions, both legal and religious, can help in alleviating fears and concerns about the right to refuse treatment.
    - *Training* This is important so that health care professionals can deal with the increasing requests of patients who may be displeased with certain advance care available.

Nutrition and hydration

There has been considerable concern over the issue of nutrition and hydration and this therefore merits separate attention.

It is accepted that when patients choose to die at home, they may not receive the same amount of medical treatment and attention that they receive in hospital. Once in hospital hydration drips are set up and almost invariably remain there until a patient dies. When veins become thrombosis and it is difficult to find an appropriate site, the use of subcutaneous drips have become commonplace. Whilst there are difficulties in understanding whether this actually provides any benefit, and indeed it may provide discomfort when the underlying skin becomes swollen, it does provide a sense of security.

All patients are entitled to food and drink of adequate quantity and quality and to the help necessary that they need to eat and drink. If a patient refuses to eat and drink or has problems with eating or drinking, one must address the underlying physiological and psychological problems (such as mouth ulcers or depression). If a patient needs assistance, this should be provided. *If one is convinced* that a patient is not receiving adequate nutrition or hydration by mouth, even with support, one must assess their condition and consider clinically assisted nutrition and hydration.

The following points are important in this consideration (Jones, 2010):

1. A futile treatment is unethical and not in the patient's best interest
2. This treatment frequently ignores the respect to the autonomy of patients and moreover breaches the other three principles which today are considered very relevant in health care. It causes harm, it provides no good (beneficence) and it consumes resources which may otherwise benefit other patients (Justice0. It should

be stressed that the last consideration in the previous sentence, although important is not the focus of end-of-life care however.

3. This challenge is especially relevant in the nutritional support and hydration of patients toward the end-of-life.
   - For example, "the natural history of advanced dementia is commonly for cognitive decline with deterioration in swallowing, leading to malnutrition and finally death from pneumonia. Until only 30 years ago, such patients were treated permissively without artificial nutrition and hydration (ANH). However the introduction of the fine-bore nasogastric feeding tube (NGT) and percutaneous endoscopic gastrostomy (PEG) in the early 1980s meant that many demented patients could be fed artificially – frequently without proper consent. This inevitably led to considerable debate. It is now clear that the use of PEG feeding in dementia achieves no discernible benefit in most patients but often causes mortality and morbidity.
4. In other words this treatment breaches all four principles
5. The dilemma is between those who espouse the preservation of life at all costs as opposed to those who at the other extreme espouse euthanasia or assisted suicide.
6. It should be noted that non-provision of futile treatment is not in any form an assisted suicide.
7. Futile treatment should be based on evidence and scientific knowledge and not on anecdotal or opinion, especially of lay persons. Whilst communication may be difficult it is essential to explain that what one aims to achieve is the comfort of the patient and that preserving life at all costs not only does not benefit the patient but it causes considerable suffering. That religions agree on this may help health care professionals explain the rationale behind omitting futile treatment.
8. Conversely when there is disagreement, the decision should be based on a proper informed choice. Under law patients are able to refuse or consent to treatment through a proper informed consent process, requiring:
   - Information necessary for a "reasonable person standard"
   - Making sure that there is adequate understanding of goals, and outcomes

- A voluntary choice on the part of the patient
- Capacity to consent
- A decision to consent or refuse a treatment

9. Conversely patients are not able, under law, to request treatment which is proved to be futile for that particular patient – ranging from keeping people on life support systems to ANH.
10. Under normal circumstances doctors should consider nutritional support and hydration. It should be clearly understood however that such provision when death is imminent and recognised to be near, can be disproportionate and cause morbidity and suffering, especially if one has to re-insert needles, etc. In this circumstance, even if it is doubtful whether it is futile, the overall well-being of the patient should be considered. Removing an intravenous line at the end, for example, is *not* passive euthanasia. It simply acknowledges that death is the inevitable outcome and one seeks the charitable removal of disproportionate treatment or treatment which has now become extraordinary, as one seeks when administering pain relief.
11. The following quotation is put as an important guideline:
    - The concept of a distressing death by starvation or dehydration as a result of a fatal condition leads understandable to the commonly held belief that nutrition must be achieved by all means possible. This is a valid belief if the patient is able to perceive ANH as beneficial. On the other hand, if cognitive capacity is serious impaired and likely to be progressive, and if there is no potential for achieving the objective of improving duration or quality of life, no benefit can accrue from imposing ANH which would be unethical. This is particularly true for a potentially dangerous invasive procedure such as PEG. The possibility that ANH might prolong dying must always be considered. A decision not to provide nutritional support while continuing intravenous (i.v.) hydration should also be recognised as irrational since this practice also prolongs the dying process without benefit. However, if ANH might provide support during an acute episode, such as a post-cerebrovascular accident (CVA) or head injury, it is justified even if the patient is unaware."

Defined outcomes in helping overcome difficulties (Jones, 2010):

1. In most cases decisions on ANH and consent are settled without dissent but consensus cannot always be achieved.
2. In these circumstances, a 'trial of treatment' with specified and agreed objectives over a finite period of time may help clarify the correct decision regarding ANH.
3. It should be emphasized that withdrawal of treatment is held to be identical to withholding treatment morally, ethically and legally, despite the greater emotional burden on the relatives and care team associated with withdrawal of treatment.
   - This is a principle of 'moral equivalence'.
   - It should be explained clearly before and 'trial of treatment'.
   - Starting treatment never means that a treatment ought to be continued, especially if it is considered futile, extraordinary or in any way disproportionate.
4. Defining the outcomes:
   - One should actively ask, "does this patient need nutritional support?" or "does this patient need a PEG?" or even, "do we need to re-insert a needle to provide an i.v. line?"
   - These are pertinent questions and should be answered *clinically* before any discussion. Such decision should not be taken empirically.
   - In case of an advanced care plan, nutritional support is never an emergency and one can provide hydration to allow time to determine any prior decision by the patient.
   - If ANH is considered potentially futile, then its provision is unethical. It simply prolongs morbidity and even suffering.
   - Defined outcomes should include:
     - Prevention of malnutrition
     - Pneumonia and bed sores
     - Improvement in quality of life
     - Length of survival.
   - In regard to ii and iv, one should consider pain relief without actually providing a support which would simply prolong a natural process.
   - In cases of dementia, since there is little or no evidence to support the achievement of any of these objectives using

artificial nutritional support, ANH is potentially futile and therefore unethical treatment which is capable of greater harm. Instead, it is recommended that careful feeding be offered despite the risk of aspiration pneumonia (Jones, 2010)

The following are relevant points in a clinical decision process regarding ANH:

1. In many laws nutrition and hydration provided by a drip or tube are regarded in law as medical treatment, and should therefore be treated in the same way as other medical interventions.
2. However many consider this treatment as basic and it is important to listen to the patients and those close to them, including their cultural and religious beliefs, whilst explaining the issues including benefits, risks and burdens, as described above.
3. If you consider ANH to be inappropriate and there is no consensus, you have a right to objection of conscience and follow the guidelines provided in this document in this regard.
4. If a patient lacks capacity but you judge, notwithstanding the patient is in the end stage of the disease, that death is not bound to occur within hours or days, then you must provide clinically assisted nutrition or hydration if it would be of overall benefit to them.
5. One should continue to monitor and assess and not hesitate to withdraw treatment if it is not considered to provide overall benefit. The patient's interests must be thoroughly considered.
6. If there is consensus that ANH need not be started or ought to be withdrawn, one must still make sure that the patient is comfortable and any distressing symptoms addressed.
7. Recognition of death:
   - If a patient is expected to die within hours or days, and you consider that the burdens and risks outweigh any benefits which treatment may provide, then it is unethical to start or continue with this treatment. ANH must be considered *separately*, but in the same manner.
   - The patient's condition must be kept under review especially if they live longer than you expected. In this case the benefits and risks must be reassessed again.

DNACPR – Do Not Attempt Cardio-Pulmonary Resuscitation

This document does not attempt to re-write the document on DNACPR at Mater Dei Hospital. The intention is to emphasise some points, some of which are already mentioned in said document.

1. Every person who is not approaching death has a right to CPR. When death is imminent one has to define whether by imminence one is meaning over the next few months or is in hospital and expecting to die. In the former case CPR can be considered unless there is a clinical reason or a directive not to.
2. DNACPR documents have to be re-visited during each ward round as the situation of the patient may change
3. They should be discussed with the patient and relatives if possible but when death is considered imminent, it is the medical team which should make the final decision.
4. It should be kept in mind that a futile CPR will keep the person alive and in agony simply to wait for another similar episode.
5. CPR may be successful by restarting a heartbeat, breathing and restoring circulation. These benefits must be weighed against the burdens and risks and should be discussed sensitively if patients and relatives are prepared to talk. Discussion should not be forced as people may understand that one has given up on them or on their loved one. One must provide accurate assessment of the burdens including the risk that one CPR may lead to another in a short while.
6. In patients who lack capacity, CPR must be discussed with the legal proxy. If there is no legal proxy one must discuss with those who are close to the patient and give them the same details as described in point 5.
7. If relatives or the proxy insist on CPR and as the responsible physician you still consider it would not be for the overall benefit of the patient, you should explain your reasoning (for example that it will burden the patient and cause futile distress) and explain to them their right for a second opinion.
8. DNACPR applies only to CPR and in no way should it imply that the patient does not receive other treatments, including other extraordinary treatment which at the time is being given. Such statements as "this patient is on a DNACPR order" which

is meant to imply to a visiting on-call doctor not to give some other form of treatment is be avoided. Clinical information provided must be factual and non-directive.

9. Until such time as Advance Care Plans are in place, a person re-admitted to hospital who was formerly on a DNACPR order, should be re-evaluated and the decision must include any improvement the patient has made.

Spiritual care

The following points are taken from the "Statement form the Danish Council of Ethics", Spiritual Care for the Dying (The Danish Council of Ethics, 2004):

1. Spiritual care is often used synonymously with spiritual and existential care; it includes care which is both specifically religious and regard for the existential issues and concerns that a dying person may go through.
2. On the verge of death a person may be confronted with great existential issues such as the meaning of the life lived, the loss of life and the relationship with the next-of-kin, about faith in God, and faith in life after death.
3. A person also experiences a series of agonising losses; as a result of impairment of health a person may not continue to preserve social relations and activities which before could be done.
4. Faith and religiousness are a significant aspect of many people's outlook on life. It is important to acknowledge this and not in any way diminish their outlook at these final stages as it can increase existential suffering.
5. The scope of religious care is not to triumph over death but rather to acknowledge the impotence one feels and that this is outside the power vested in any human being. Religious care helps the dying person to recognize the limits of his or her own power and to come to terms that God is taking over.
6. The Danish Council gives four examples which conclude that:
   - From a theological point of view, patients can be helped to direct the anger that life is the way it is towards God (and that He acknowledges this) as otherwise it could be directed towards the people around them and this compounds loneliness. They

may be comforted in knowing that death does brings with it a loneliness that no one can reach into. This is regarded as a 'vertical' approach of the person with God.

- From a psychological point of view it may be fear of death, desperation, anger or difficult relations with next-of-kin which may need to be addressed. The help psychologists or counsellors can provide may need to be directed not only to the dying person but also to relations which may be involved. This is a horizontal work which is complementary to the vertical described above.
- Experienced nurses have acknowledged that there may be an avoidance of contact with the dying person. Some acknowledge that this is due to the fact that nurses are trained to 'fix' things. To overcome this nurses acknowledge that it is important to establish contact and enter into a dialogue with the dying, during which the latter does not have to hold back their need to share their thoughts. This requires the nurse to show a genuine interest and that she is taking time to enter into this dialogue. Whilst they should recognise that the patient may express frustration about living and dying, one should be opportunistic and recognise points where they can offer some assistance, such as communion, or speaking with a spiritual person. The nurse can also be a means of conveying messages such as that of a mother who is disappointed that she will not see her child grow into a teenager; the nurse can convey this worry to the person concerned.
- Finally the doctor should not think of themselves only as a 'medical technician' but a 'medical humanist'. Although doctor's contacts with patients are relatively short, they can be very intense and have a special role to play in spiritual and existential suffering. Every word the doctor utters remains in the patient's recollection, being turned over and over. It is primarily the doctor who speaks about the progression of the disease. It is important to build trust in order to foster confidence. The doctor can encourage the patient to do certain things now rather than postpone if he or she feels that the time is short. Conversely the patient must give meaning

to the time ahead, if one is envisaging a longer period. This helps the patient talk about "the whole point of being here". Indirectly these messages point to the patient the length of time left. Pointing out a sort holiday or getting important things done is quite different than encouraging one to take long holidays and doing all the things that they always wanted to do. Although the doctor may not be the right person to provide specialised spiritual care, one should show willingness and ability to take spiritual care seriously. Experience shows that both the patient and the next-of-kin often request a talk with the doctor despite having been thoroughly informed about the disease.

7. Ethical considerations
   - There should be respect for the patient's self determination.
   - One should explain that pain can be relieved by pain relief and explain that ethically this is permissible.
   - Spiritual care should be offered if the patient feels the illness is a punishment from God.
   - It is important for the health professional to be versant with the main spiritual declarations of different religions, and especially the Catholic religion in the Maltese context, with regard to end-of-life. One can point out specific paragraphs of the Catechism which speak about the difference between passive euthanasia and not having to give futile, extraordinary or disproportionate treatment, and also, knowledge that providing pain relief which may hasten death follows the principle of double effect and is morally allowed.
   - The monotheistic religions (Judaism, Christianity, and Islam) all agree on these basic principles.

Bibliography and references

Abela, J., Mallia, P. (2010). An evaluation of palliative care education in the specialist training programme in family medicine. *Malta Medical Journal, 22*(04), 26-26-33.

Gawande, A. (2015). *Being Mortal. Illness, Medicine and what Matters in the End.* Wellcome Collection, London.

General Medical Council. (2010). In GMC (Ed.), *Treatment and care towards the end-of-life. good practice in decision-making.* London: General Medical Council.

Jones, B. (2010). Ethics and nutrition towards the end-of-life. *Clinical Medicine, 10*(6), 607-610.

Mallia, P., Abela, J. (2011). An evaluation of the palliative care module in the specialist training programme in family medicine. *Malta Medical Journal, 22*(4), 26-33.

Marshall, P., Robson, R. (2018) in Bioethics Education Project. (Ed.), *Conflict resolution primer.* Royal College of Physicians and Surgeons of Canada. http://www.royalcollege.ca/rcsite/documents/bioethics/conflict-resolution-summary-e.pdf

Neveroff Dubler, N. (2005). Conflict and consensus at the end-of-life. *Hasting Center Report, Special Report*, S19-S25, p S23.

Nutik Zitter, J. (2017). *Extreme Measures. Finding a Better Path to the End-of-life.* Avery, New York.

O'Mahony, S. (2016). *The Way We Die*, Head of Zeus, London.

The Danish Council of Ethics. (2004). In Danish Council of Ethics (Ed.), *End-of-life. ethical challenges and problems.*

Consulted documents

Draft guides concerning the decision-making process regarding medical treatment in end-of-life situations, Council of Europe. DH-BIO (2103), Strasbourg.

"Spiritual care for the dying", from "*End-of-life. Ethical Challenges and Problems*", The Danish council on Ethics, Copenhagen, 2004.

Treatment and Care towards the end-of-life: good practice in decision-making. General Medical Council Guidelines for Doctors, UK. 2010.

Further reading

Advance Care Planning in End-of-life Care; Thomas, K, Lobo, B. Oxford University Press, 2011.

Medical Decision-Making. A physician's guide. Schwartz, A., Bergus, G. Cambridge Medicine, Cambridge University Press, Cambridge, New York, 2008.

Pathways through care at the end-of-life. A guide to patient-centred care; Hayes, A. et al., Jessica Kingsley Publishers, 2014.

Contributors to the consensus document

Professor Kevin Aquilina, Dean, Faculty of Laws; Dr Daniela Galea; Rev. Dr Mark Sultana.

Professor Pierre Mallia, Main author and editor, Bioethics Research Programme.

Further literature

Abela, J., Mallia, P. (2016). "Maltese Doctors: views and experiences on end-of-life decisions and care", *Maltese Medical Journal,* 28(2): 16-26.

Abela, J., Mallia, P. (2016). "Training in Palliative Medicine and Maltese Doctors: A Cross Sectional Survey", *Journal of the Malta college of Family Doctors,* 5(2): 13-19.

Emmerich, N., Mallia, P., Gordijn, B., Pistoia, F. "Introduction", in Emmerich, N., Mallia, P., Gordijn, B., Pistoia, F. (eds.) *Contemporary European Perspective on the Ethics of End-of-life Care, accepted for publication by Springer-Nature, due 2018*

Mallia, P., "Stressors in the elderly population in Malta – advanced care planning and taking care of grandchildren", in *Active and healthy Aging in Malta,* Formosa, Martin (ed.), due 2018, University of Malta, *in progress.*

Mallia, P. (2018). "A practical comparison between Islamic and Christian moral guidelines towards harmonization of end-of-life care", *submitted to International Journal of Bioethics, Ed. Christian Byk.* JAHR. 9. 185-203. 10.21860/j.9.2.3.

Mallia, P., "Does Betty Higden live on? Dickens's Contribution to Gerontology Today", in *Journal of the International Institute on Ageing,* United Nations, 2014 (4): 23-25.

Mallia, P. "Development and status of Bioethics in Malta", in *Compendium and Atlas of Global Bioethics*, Henk Ten Have & Bert Gordijn (eds.), Springer, 2012.

Mallia, P., "Are clarifications of feeding and hydration in PVS needed by Catholic authorities?", *International Journal of Bioethics*, 2012, 23(3-4): 179-188.

Mallia, P., "Gender issues and the elderly: are working parents affecting negatively the Maltese elderly population?", in *Bold: United Nations Journal of the International Institute on Ageing*, 2012: 22(2); 2-6.

Mallia, P., "Clinical Intervention in Aging: Ethico-legal issues in assessing risk and benefit", *Journal of Clinical Intervention in Aging*, 2010:5; 373-380.

Mallia, P., "Biopsychosocial and End-of-Life Care – timely intervention for Elderly", *Journal of the International Institute on Aging*, 2010: 20(4); 22-29.

Mallia, P., *You and Your Doctor*, Agenda Publishers, Malta 2006.

Mallia, P., "Advancing Advanced Directives", in *Bold, Journal of the UN Institute on aging*, Vol. 15, No. 2, 2005: 27-30.

Mallia, P., "Advance Directives", M. Cauchi (ed), *Bioethical Issues at the Beginning and End-of-life*, Bioethics Consultative Committee, Malta, 2002: 135-140.

Mallia, P., *The Beginning and End-of-life. Moral Controversy*, PEG Publishers, Malta, 2002.

Mallia, P. Abela, J., Abela, M. (2017) "Harmonisation of End-of-life care – a summer school to help health care professionals to identify strengths and weaknesses in end-of-life care in their setting" submitted to International Journal of Ethics Education.

Mallia, P., Abela, J., "*An evaluation of the Palliative Care Module in the Specialist Training Programme in Family Medicine*", in Maltese Medical Journal, 2010: 22(4): 26-33.

Mallia, P., Abela, J. "Chapter 17. Developing a curriculum towards pathways to improve end-of-life care and Advanced Care Planning in specific setting", in *Harmonising End-of-life Care. An European Union Project.* Mallia, P., Gordijn, B., Pistoia, F., Emmerich, N. (eds.) to be submitted to Wiley Publishers.

Mallia, P., Gordijn, B., Pistoia, F., Emmerich, N., "Introduction. Harmonisation of the end-of-life in local situations", in *Harmonising*

End-of-life Care. An European Union Project. Mallia, P., Gordijn, B., Pistoia, F., Emmerich, N. (eds.) to be submitted to Wiley publishers.

Mallia, P., Gordijn, B., Pistoia, F., Emmerich, N.,*"The Future and Conclusions"* in *Harmonising End-of-life Care. An European Union Project.* Mallia, P., Gordijn, B., Pistoia, F., Emmerich, N. (eds.) to be submitted to Wiley Publishers.

Laws

The Constitution of Malta.

European Convention Act, Chapter 319 of the Laws of Malta.

Health Care Professions Act, Chapter 464 of the Laws of Malta.

Mental Health Act, Chapter 525 of the Laws of Malta.

Reflective note
Thinking about the elderly

One of the first responses to the COVID-19 pandemic was a proportionate lockdown.[1] As a general practitioner, what struck me most in the following months was the unappreciated vulnerability of the elderly. Many stayed inside due of fear; others ventured on as if nothing were happening (also a reflection of vulnerability); still others were restricted either because of their physical ailments or because they were in homes. We need to take stock, learn from experiences and think out a plan which would help the elderly and those looking after them cope better since the future is still unclear.

Whilst the generosity of society was indeed felt, with groceries and medicines being delivered to door, those living in flats also had some comfort in each other. However, fear and for others loneliness crept slowly on many and as doctors we had to deal with depressions and stress. The media certainly played its important part many found much comfort in the daily mass. Many appreciated the archbishop for his simplicity, short and to-the-point homilies, and his devotion to the cause. Television can play an important role of communication. 6.30pm programmes for children are not; children have social media today. We coped as much as we could. Of course, we made mistakes. This was and continues to be a learning process. But now is time for some reflective practice.

For example, a patient in a home had to be sent to hospital three times in the first three months. Each time he recovered he was sent to the Msida home for two weeks' quarantine. The people there were nice but the place had no internet with the 87-year-old used to communicate with his family and also to pass the time. The tragedy was that it all

[1] Published in *The Malta Independent on Sunday*, January 2020.

was in vain. The home was locked down as the virus became endemic. People were transferred. Foreign care workers living in tight quarters with many others working in different environments were coming and going into these homes – perhaps hotel accommodation on a longer-term basis can be arranged for these people, whom we are too quick to blame.

It would be appropriate that government and NGOs get together to formulate coherent plans. We can learn a lot even by listening to the people who work in these places. When I visited one of these homes to see patients, I noticed increased depressed states, worrying, anxiety, anger at not being able to leave the room to go even to the common areas to chat and of course the reduced visits from relatives. In one instance anger and confusion turned to violence with severe bruising to the victim. Perhaps we need to note which signs were on the rise and how we can help people to cope. Perhaps it is time to integrate primary mental health into primary care in a coherent manner. Although in fairness an attempt was done by the Minister for Health, this was with regard to follow-up on patients and not actually primary care. Another attempt involving a re-thinking of pathways will help primary care physicians cope and be ready for mental health issues in such current situations. Clearly it was the elderly who suffered the most in this regard. Private family doctors can involve community nurses, health care workers and if need be psychologists to be in touch regularly with patients, even if by telephone, if they are given the appropriate support.

On a wider scheme one has to assess prevention rather than cure. Locally the health minister would have had the airports shut down immediately. Prof. Gauci and was right when she said that the virus could have been avoided in Malta. What is more concerning is how the WHO did not use the *Precautionary Principle* when there were enough red flags showing the danger of the virus when it was still in China. Whilst it is true that the WHO guidelines to countries for pandemics is showing solidarity, interpreting solidarity, as always is tricky. Many heard with incredulity the WHO transmission basically saying that the virus is not understood, there will be a pandemic, people will die, but we need to show solidarity. The advice was to keep airports open! Is this the role of WHO? The later it supported shuts downs. Many people were asking why allow it to happen deliberately? People lose faith in organisations this way. As a matter of fact, the EU countries in imminent danger ignored the same EU advice to concur with the WHO. Later precautionary measures followed suit. We did show solidarity with each other notwithstanding the closing of borders. Nobody suffered any hunger. I am quite certain that this will not be the first virus we will have to deal with. Whilst no one can judge decisions in good faith; people will judge our future actions.

The maxim taught about elders is 'more life to years than years to life'. Although encouraged to leave home for daily walks, many were overwhelmed by fear, and some simply could not. Together we can find ways to make their lives better. For example, short visits from relatives using the usual precautions can be encouraged. We used alcohol, used masks, social distance making short frequent visits. We can also help them to go out for walks if they cannot. Conversely, we hardly have an option to keep our teens inside – more input from education is needed here. They hardly practice social distancing, and we know it. So, allowing some slack for the elderly is possible. The social burden of our elderly rests on us – the answer cannot be isolation – especially in homes. This is not public health any longer but the health *of* the public one (more on this in a future article), when utilitarian measure have to move to a more principled and individual approach.

Looking at a more positive angle, this global 'warning' has given us a breath of fresh air showing us how clear our waters and skies could be, how much less traffic we can have by using the technology we have at our disposal. We suddenly did away with a lot of paperwork when just a few months before people were complaining to me that they had to go in person to deliver a form for a driving licence renewal.

Index